Binocular Vision

Binocular Vision: An Inquiry into Psychoanalytic Techniques and Field Theory explains field theory from a Bionian perspective, while exploring the relationship between art and psychoanalysis.

Elena Molinari starts from Bion's double definition to explore the relationship between the conscious and unconscious thought process. She looks at a wide range of specific situations where field theory can be beneficial, from mother-baby therapy with a borderline mother, couple and group therapy, and the relationship of female subjectivity between an analyst and an adolescent analysand. In each situation, Molinari unpicks what Binocular Vision might mean as a transformative process used to explore the primitive parts of the mind. By doing so, she brings the reader back to the earliest developments of the primary relationship between analyst and client, and how this process can unite the psychoanalytic process and the artistic process.

The book has been written for psychotherapists approaching and utilising field theory in child and adult psychoanalysis, and offers vital knowledge to clinicians working with patients in primitive states.

Elena Molinari is a psychoanalyst at Italian Psychoanalytic Society and an International Psychoanalytical Association member. She began her professional life working as a paediatrician. She has worked as a private analyst with adults, children and adolescents. Currently she is teaching Child Neuropsychiatry for the postgraduate course in Art Therapy at Brera Accademia di Belle Arti in Milan.

"In this book, the psychoanalyst Elena Molinari presents her refined psychoanalytic thought and her keen sensitivity built up over the course of her career, which began in medicine (paediatrics) and reached psychoanalysis and art. The concepts of Bion, and of Antonino Ferro and collaborators, are developed through clinical reports and chapters on artists and their works. Reading the book provides a rich opportunity to study contemporary psychoanalytic theory and technique articulated with aesthetics."

Alexandre Martins de Mello, Brazilian psychoanalyst and psychiatrist

"In her thought-provoking book, Elena Molinari delves into the intriguing concept of binocular vision in psychoanalysis, providing a fresh and comprehensive perspective on this essential topic. By skillfully navigating through various realms, from psychoanalytic theory to philosophy, she presents a compelling argument for the transformative power of binocular vision. Drawing from her extensive experience as a psychoanalyst and pediatrician, and through captivating case studies and theoretical insights, Molinari demonstrates how this dual system of reference unlocks the depths of the analytic process, illuminating the dynamics of traumas and facilitating healing. The book goes beyond the therapeutic setting to explore how art and psychoanalysis intersect. The author skillfully weaves together the works of influential figures like Bion, Beckett, and Rothko, highlighting the profound connection between creativity, powerlessness, and therapeutic transformation. This groundbreaking work challenges traditional notions of analytic practice and offers innovative tools for the psychoanalytic community. The author's adept use of diverse disciplines and her ability to synthesize complex concepts make *Binocular Vision: An Inquiry into Psychoanalytic Techniques and Field Theory* a valuable resource for both practitioners and researchers alike. Its unique perspective and interdisciplinary approach breathe new life into psychoanalysis and leave a lasting impact on our understanding of the human psyche and its capacity to transform."

Giuseppe Civitarese, author of *Psychoanalytic Field Theory: A Contemporary Introduction* (Routledge)

"In this riveting collection of linked essays exploring the complex dynamics of psychic reciprocity, Molinari harnesses her intimate appreciation of art to illuminate the movements of experiencing, meaning-making, and transformation as they emerge in a multitude of clinical settings. Gem-like vignettes capture the inspired work of a creative healer."

Wendy W. Katz, Assistant Clinical Professor of Medical Psychology (in Psychiatry), Columbia University Medical Center, and Training and Supervising Analyst, Columbia University Psychoanalytic Center, New York, USA

Binocular Vision

An Inquiry into Psychoanalytic Techniques and Field Theory

Elena Molinari

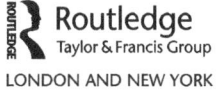

Routledge
Taylor & Francis Group

LONDON AND NEW YORK

Designed cover image: Cover image from ETRU, National Etruscan Museum of Villa Giulia under the CC-BY 3.0 license. Hydria with blinding of Polyphemus and pursuit of Deianira and Nessus by Heracles, Cerveteri, Necropolis of Banditaccia, tomb 1, 530–520 BC. See https://www.museoetru.it/termini-duso

First published 2024
by Routledge
4 Park Square, Milton Park, Abingdon, Oxon OX14 4RN

and by Routledge
605 Third Avenue, New York, NY 10158

Routledge is an imprint of the Taylor & Francis Group, an informa business

© 2024 Elena Molinari

British Library Cataloguing-in-Publication Data
A catalogue record for this book is available from the British Library

Library of Congress Cataloging-in-Publication Data
Names: Molinari, Elena, 1960– author.
Title: Binocular vision in psychoanalysis / Elena Molinari.
Description: Abingdon, Oxon ; New York, NY : Routledge, 2024. | Includes bibliographical references and index.
Identifiers: LCCN 2023027676 (print) | LCCN 2023027677 (ebook) | ISBN 9781032483986 (hardback) | ISBN 9781032478968 (paperback) | ISBN 9781003388838 (ebk)
Subjects: LCSH: Psychoanalysis. | Psychoanalysis and art. | Binocular vision—Psychological aspects. | Field theory (Social psychology) | Psychotherapist and patient.
Classification: LCC RC506 .M65 2024 (print) | LCC RC506 (ebook) | DDC 616.89/17—dc23/eng/20230817
LC record available at https://lccn.loc.gov/2023027676
LC ebook record available at https://lccn.loc.gov/2023027677

ISBN: 978-1-032-48398-6 (hbk)
ISBN: 978-1-032-47896-8 (pbk)
ISBN: 978-1-003-38883-8 (ebk)

DOI: 10.4324/9781003388838

Typeset in Times New Roman
by Apex CoVantage, LLC

A Paolo,
con cui ho pensato, discusso e vissuto in modo
"binoculare."

Contents

Introduction

What does binocular vision mean in psychoanalysis? There is no reference to the ophthalmological medical use of the term or to the opposition between principles in Eastern philosophies. To start defining the topic, I could explain what is meant by binocular in a psychoanalytic setting (laboratory). Psychoanalysis grapples with the dilemma of not being able to be a science while striving to be a cure, and it oscillates, between seeking scientific evidence or metrics and pursuing empirical efficacy.

Could the Grubbs's test,[1] which involves comparing laboratory results with two other controls, serve as an analogous model for scientific measurements in psychoanalysis?

In psychoanalytic therapy, the therapist-patient pair or therapist-group dyad constitutes the experimental situation. It was precisely within a therapy group context that the concept of *binocular vision,* introduced by Bion, emerged as a transformative act in working with patients. I have been reflecting on the sessions I conducted with groups of supervised therapist colleagues over the past few years. The method involved reading two sessions presented without anamnestic data, after which the associations that arose in the group were examined by the supervising analyst in relation to the group dynamics that were unfolding.

This dual system of reference, or binocular vision, has proven to be a powerful tool for gaining insight into the less accessible areas of the mind – those where unrepressed traumas lie, the experiences that have caused significant disruptions in psychic development and the psychotic aspects in general of the personality.

While one supervision in particular is elaborated upon in detail in the final chapter of this book, Chapter 11, the concept of binocular vision permeates all of the preceding chapters. This book does not consist of a collection of psychoanalytic cases but rather is an attempt to define new tools within the psychoanalytic laboratory.

Drawing inspiration from the book *The Art of Fielding*, which explores how binocular vision is essential in the context of playing defence in baseball, I became interested in examining how binocular vision manifests in the construction of relational fields in which there is no one subject who possesses knowledge and another who lacks it. The post-Bionian field theory research, developed by Baranger, Ferro,

DOI: 10.4324/9781003388838-1

Civitarese and others, focuses on the relationship and encounters between the conscious and unconscious aspects of both the patient and the analyst. Within this theoretical framework, experiments have been attempted and reported in Chapter 9, both within the analyst's mind and in the setting and process of psychoanalysis.

Chapters 1 and 3 highlight the crucial role that children can play in helping their mothers or parents explore their psychic difficulties, which are often the root of developmental issues to some extent. This perspective stems from my training and extensive practice as a paediatrician, which allows me to observe problematic family situations through an analytical gaze.

The *Odyssey* of transgenerational traumas can make patients and analysts blind (Chapter 7). The binocular vision experiments try to observe *the inaccessible unconscious*[2] of these difficulties with children (Chapter 10), in couple's lives (Chapter 5) and in personal symptoms (Chapter 7).

Chapter 10 presents several short cases that illustrate how much we can learn from children themselves, their persistent attempts to connect with their parents even in the face of evident difficulties. Being able to adopt a binocular view of these life situations, merging medical and analytical practices, has cultivated this unique perspective.

As I write this introduction, I realise how I have structured the chapters by placing the experiences that shaped my current thinking towards the end, while opening with the most daring reversal that constituted the book's objective: a focus on child creativity and the therapeutic implications that can result from it. Binocular vision undoubtedly has transformative implications not only for patients but also for analysts.

Chapter 4 exemplifies the parallel emergence of subjectification in a young adolescent and the redefinition of the analyst's role.

In Chapter 5, I recount the story of a couple seeking therapy for a profound relationship crisis. The journey to self-discovery required embracing two distinct perspectives, and I drew inspiration from the stages of Ulysses's journey back to Ithaca to provide an imaginative backdrop. In other words, couple therapy can be seen as a particular application of binocular vision.

Chapter 8 delves into how this way of thinking spills over into the therapeutic setting. It challenges the notion that the number of sessions or the use of the couch alone can define analytic practice. Instead, adopting a binocular view of the setting, the measure for a good course can be "comfort" – a practical analogue of what Bion referred to as being *in unison with the patient's mind*.

Finally, I reflect upon the topic of art. During a conference, Massimo Cacciari contemplated Hegel's statement that "thought and reflection have surpassed the domain of fine art"[3] and concluded that contemporary art and artists work with the means of ineffectiveness. He cited Beckett and Bacon as examples. In my first book, I added a third "B" to this equation: Wilfred Bion. I explored how analysts could reflect on themselves and their powerless impotence.

Teaching at the Brera Academy of Fine Arts for many years has allowed me to engage in intense exchanges of thoughts, emotions and inspirations with young artists. The research within the academy aimed to transcend Kant's dilemma of art, which can no longer express the sublime. Only through experiment after experiment, research after research, transformation after transformation, without arriving at a self-satisfied art, the artist must work with means of ineffectiveness, Kant 1781.[4] Bion also reflected on Kant, almost to the point of being labelled a neo-Kantian, deviating from the Freudian dogmatism prevalent in the psycho-analytic community at that time. Bion was Beckett's analyst, a fact that Beckett conveyed in several of his novels, such as Murphy.[5] Together, they embarked on a quest to develop a method of reflection on powerlessness and fragility, driven by Beckett's fragile and creative mind. To some extent, I continue along this line of thought, studying how beautiful art can be therapeutic. Not consolatory, thera-peutic, because Bionian techniques are as intricate and complex as theoretical physics, hence the shared terminology of "field," "alpha" and "beta elements." And like a patient scientist, the analyst folds and unfolds, like origami, the space that separates them from the patient, as I had illustrated in a chapter of my first book,[6] drawing inspiration from the story of Japanese engineer Koryo Miura, who transformed the ancient art of paper folding into an innovative method for folding the photovoltaic cells of spaceships.

In the present book, the dialogue with art becomes explicit, particularly in Chapters 2 and 6. In Chapter 2, I recount how art exercises I conducted years ago to refine tactile sensitivity aided in establishing contact with a child on the autism spectrum. It not only allowed me to connect with him but also provided glimpses into the cognitive processes through which his mind sought to bring order to expe-rience. In Chapter 6, I compare Bion and Rothko, two contemporaries who likely remained unaware of each other's existence and research. Despite their vastly different realms, they exhibit intriguing points of intersection. In the last part of his life, particularly during the seminar he delivered in Paris in 1979, Bion encap-sulated his research by offering the listener an aesthetic experience, rather than presenting it in a purely theoretical manner. This experience, in therapy, needs to be dreamed and mentalised, becoming a conscious and unconscious experience simultaneously. It is the product of binocular vision, both within the patient and between the patient and the analyst.

Jean Paul Sartre[7] wrote about the method, stating, "So the image as image is describable only by a second-order act, in which the look is turned away from the object and directed at the way in which the object is given. It is this reflective act that permits the judgment: 'I have an image'. It is necessary to repeat here what has been known since Descartes: a reflective consciousness delivers us absolutely certain data."

Furthermore, we can incorporate the concept of binocular vision to acknowledge the certainty of our limited understanding or recognition of what we do not yet know.

Echoing Robert Coles, I would conclude by saying: "We work in the dark, we do what we can, we give what we have; our doubt is our passion, and our passion is our task. The rest is the madness of art."[8]

Notes

1 Grubbs 1950.
2 Bion 1997b.
3 Hegel 1975.
4 Cited from the transcription of a conference of Massimo Cacciari in Milano 2009 Feb (Sequeri 2009).
5 Beckett, *Murphy*, Einaudi, 1980.
6 E. Molinari 2017.
7 Sartre 2004.
8 From the introduction of Robert Coles (Lehman 1999).

Chapter 1

Turning the roles upside down

Can a baby dream the mother's infantile trauma?

The *open field* in psychoanalytic literature is an expression that calls to mind the observational aspect of the relational model[1] and non-linear dynamics systems theory.[2] At the same time, in spoken language, it refers to the need to keep ourselves open to discovering the unexpected. The *field* concept also has something of its original roots in theoretical physics, namely, the need for tools and a clear enough theoretical frame to put some order into observations.

Bion created the grid (of the field) as a tool for observing and categorising the transformations in the analytical setting. He also described how sensory elements could move through rows and columns towards mentalisation. Conversely, in neuroscience, the *open field* is an experimental tool used to study animal behaviour in response to different stimuli. It consists of a box with a grid at the bottom and a video camera at the top. Video recordings allow investigators to observe animals' free movements and the frequency of their freezing episodes in response to traumatic events. Findings reveal that if stressor events occur in early development or repeatedly over time, they can interfere with the endocrine system and the growth of the hippocampus, a region of the brain that plays a crucial role in learning, memory, and the integration of emotional and cognitive systems.

Although observing body and movements using grids in an *open field* in neuroscience and psychoanalysis belongs to very different theoretical models, it represents the starting point of a therapeutic experiment. It consists of focusing on the developing healthy sensation of a baby to help a borderline mother become more conscious of her raw and unmodulated feelings emerging from the body. The baby helped the mother and the analyst too to focus on the multidimensional flow that characterises the internal dialogue between body and mind and contributes in a crucial way to the development of the ability to experience feelings and to think in the presence of emotion.

The relationship between beta and alpha elements and the centrality of the body in the primitive mental state

Between rows A (alpha elements) and B (beta elements) Bion placed the first transformation between the concrete body and the first abstraction of thought. Beta

DOI: 10.4324/9781003388838-2

elements are raw emotions and sensations expressed through the body, while alpha elements are affective pictograms representing the first step of the transformative process towards dreaming and thinking. Later, Bion changed how he first conceived of beta elements and came to regard them as more than non-mental elements; even if the direction towards mentalisation is the most important in development, beta elements may be seen as something good and necessary to mental life. Bion's thinking remains consistent with the psychoanalytic perspective of Freud and Klein, who considered emotions of a corporeal nature as the first driving elements of mental functioning. Consciousness is connected to the sensory organs, and this is the first stepping stone towards mental life. The vitality of sensations can be an important element in making the baby feel active and alive before and beyond the primitive functioning of the mind. Beta elements also have a strong tendency to evolve and withstand mental attacks.

In *Elements of Psychoanalysis*[3] Bion affirmed that beta elements were "the matrix of the mind". Although beta elements are mostly referred to as " accretions of stimuli" fit for evacuation and projection, Bion thought of them as the basic building blocks of experience, representing the hypothetical "stem cells" of experience.[4]

They occur in the immediacy of engagement with another, prior to representation in the mind, forming non-conscious analogical traces, affective contours emerging from the processes of interaction itself. So, the line that separates alpha and beta elements is closer to a contact barrier than a wall. Antonino Ferro's notion of "balpha" elements underlines that there might not always be a clear distinction between alpha and beta elements as is often described. They exist even if they cannot be used for thinking.[5]

In another but similar way, Grotstein described alpha and beta elements as being in a more fluid relationship; he formalised this idea of their dynamic relationship, transforming the line between them into a double arrow.[6] If beta or *balpha* elements represent the non-conscious analogical trace, is it possible to think about these experiences as a proto-container or the feature of an *impersonal emergent other*?[7]

The proto-container and container-contained relationship

In Bion's theory, the container is the mental space where beta elements are transformed into alpha elements. The container is a construct that arises on the border between body and mind, and which is the reason for interest in the clinical situation described here. Bion hypothesised that the baby's container would improve through the mother's capacity to take in and contain the baby's projections and then make sense of them through her maternal reverie. The restitution of more elaborated elements allows the baby to get used to them as food for his mind and develop his own container function.[8] According to Bionian theory, the relationship between container-contained is not only a primitive level of psychic functioning at the very beginning of life but a basic mechanism of any transformation, one of the functions responsible for the evolution of an element in the grid from one square to the other. In this perspective, the relationship between container and contained is not only an evolutionary function but something in oscillation at different levels of development.

Container function starts with the problem of psychic containment, but his statement that it is emotions at the body-mind interface that are at the core of the matter to transform through container/content tools reminds us that the concept remains at the border between body and mind. Moreover, Bion specifies that maternal reveries return the baby's transformed emotions through bodily actions. His description creates a precious link between body and mind, placing them in a state of oscillation from the beginning of life to adulthood.

The paradox of the container/content relationship resides in its condition of reciprocity: something that contains and something that is contained mutually take on the function of containing and being contained. From the evolutionary point of view, this means that the breast, as container of the anxieties of the newborn, can also become the opposite; the newborn can also function as a container for some aspects of the mother's personality.

In the clinical context, this reciprocity is strongly emphasised: "The key resides in the observation of the fluctuations that at a given moment put the analyst in unison with ♀ and analyzing it in unison with ♂, and in the next moment they turn the roles upside down."[9]

In the context of a wider intersubjective relationship such as in mother-baby therapy, this last observation allows us to imagine an analytic field in which beta and alpha, container/content are fluid elements in oscillation between themselves and between the subjects in the session.

It sometimes happens that the baby is on the receiving end of the mother's anxieties. However, as long as the burden does not exceed the baby's capacity and is not a too frequent occurrence, the baby can go on to develop his own container function undamaged. The drive for physical survival and the need for object relations are spontaneously and unconsciously interwoven to create a psychophysical scheme structured as an envelope. Sometime trauma rips open even the most well-sealed container, and it happens rather frequently when the mother's container is a fragile one.

The difficulties of delivery, taking care of the newborn, and affective distance from the partner who cannot accept the depression and the strange behavior make the situation a trigger to reactivate the trauma. Mother cannot use her container function for herself and the baby, but her proto-container cannot be destroyed. Cartwright[10] described the role of the proto-container as necessary in the development of the quality of internal objects, and it goes on to have an essential role in adult interactions: the proto-container catches the pre-symbolic activity and puts the expectations concerning what happened in the present moment. The analyst can then work at the cross-road of baby and mother expectations creating a contact between the healthy proto-container of the baby and the mother's damaged one. This type of work has something in common with Winnicott's concept of regression to dependence and some differences. In Winnicott, going back to dependence means to put a patient in a situation that leads him to discard his defenses and return to a position that existed before the trauma and the construction of his defenses. What is similar is repairing and restoring the mental functions starting from the point of rupture. The difference is that using pre-symbolic communication and the body is not the opposite of the mind but an important intersubjective relational tool.[11] To use the entangled fantasies contained in gestures and the movements of all the subjects in the relational field could be a way to repair the proto-container and then the damaged container.

Points of contact and difference in the healthy and pathological use of the body to communicate

Starting from his early work, Bion focused on the development of the mind from the body and the primitive level of mental functioning; he suggested a new version of the relationship between beta and alpha elements, considering them not only in a linear development. In Bion's words, there is a transitional area between rows A and B, "a series of grids repeating itself as a helix," useful to investigate the deep dialogue between bodily and mental facts.[12]

He widened his initial interest in using the body to explore the area between "corporeal fact and psychic fact" in psychotic patients.[13] In these patients, Bion hypothesised the existence of an apparatus of a bodily kind, unable to transform sensory elements in mental experience.

He shifted his interest from the link between subjects to the connection between thought and emotion in the mind. From a clinical point of view, this vertex shift allows us to treat patients with severe dissociations and broad areas of a-symbolic functioning.

What happens in the analytic setting when there is a psychotic mother who uses bodily sensations to create a "place" – as Ogden wrote[14] – in which to have experiences of herself and a baby who are both using the same sensations to create the first experience of mental life? They are using the body with its sensations and raw emotions similarly and differently simultaneously.

In the earliest phases of individual development, the child is normally dominated by motor and sensory functions, and these are the first complex phenomena of the organisation of the mind. Next, the baby uses projective identification to study his own sensations through the effect they produce on the personality into which he has projected them.

On the contrary, in a disturbed patient, the body can sometimes be used as a defense against the sorrow caused by thinking and against an "ontological anxiety".[15] The agonising early breakdown is unthinkable, inexperienced and unrepresented. It is hidden in what Bion named the inaccessible unconscious.[16] Bion and Winnicott described this deep level of unrepressed unconscious underlying the difference in intensity of feeling: Winnicott speaks about "the unthinkable"[17] and Bion of "catastrophic emotional explosion".[18] This intensity is related to the extent of the traumatisation and the failure of not being held and contained. It also depends on the time and how early the trauma occurred. The early trauma breaks the personality that forms at the beginning of the individual's life. It has already happened, but since it has not yet been experienced, it cannot get into the past tense.[19] It follows that the use of projective identification into the body of the other sometimes becomes essential for managing sensory pressures. Verbal communications are often not helpful for a baby and a disturbed mother. Psychotic patients tend to refuse symbolic communications because of the pain associated with the inability of the mind to use them. The baby needs verbal communication that is strictly linked with body communication. Verbal interpretations are all but ineffective. The reverie function, the concept of container – in the context of the container/container relationship – to be in oneness,[20] has an essential role in driving and organising experiences of a preverbal nature. The psychoanalyst has to sift through personal sensorial involvement. Thoughts reveal their relevance when they have been able to become a corpuscular matter that flows in the veins and tissues of the body, ready to contribute to the genesis of new thought in the wake of the solicitations induced by the present experience.

So, what better carrier of effective nonverbal communication than a baby?

The mother-baby therapy

The past 50 years have seen the development of several different methods of treating children's difficulties in relation to those of their parents. These methods attribute different roles to parents and babies and propose different focuses in the therapeutic process. Some authors focus specifically on the inner world of the infant and mothers, while others emphasise support for parental function. Nearly all therapists attribute a crucial role to the child, agreeing that the child's nonverbal communication can improve the process. However, they have different positions in answer to whether the child is a patient who participates in the transformation process or merely the recipient. In other words, is the child a subject capable of communicating his conscious and unconscious needs to the therapist, or is he a catalyst that feeds or fuels the therapeutic process in the mother?

The answer has consequences for both theory and technique.[21] In the first case, the therapist shares the baby's unconscious pain and speaks directly to him. In the second, the baby's suffering is regarded as the result of the mother's conflict. The analyst must connect her unconscious traumatic memories – what Fraiberg[22] called the "ghost in the nursery" – with the child's symptoms.

The request to treat an intensely distressed mother presented an opportunity to explore a different pathway within the theoretical framework of the post-Bionian psychoanalytic field.

The ethical duty and responsibility remained firm: a therapeutic responsibility to manage a borderline mother who uses bodily sensations to create a "place" in which she experiences herself and a baby who uses the same feelings to develop her first experience of mental life. They are using the body and its sensations in a way that is both similar and different.

In almost every clinical report focusing on the mother-baby interaction and the therapeutic relationship, it is the more developed subject that tries to promote the development of the less evolved one through actions, reverie and words. The hypothesis explored in this paper is the possibility that in some cases, the dynamic may be reversed. Nobody is more in touch with bodily sensations than a baby, and there is no bodily relationship closer than that within the mother-baby dyad.[23]

The case study discussed herein refers to therapy with a mother and child. The analyst attempted to make use of the baby's bodily communication, as an aesthetic gestalt, to improve the mother's mental functioning. To better describe how the baby could be a carrier of emerging meaning, we have to go back to Bion's concept of the "selected fact". Bion described it as an idea that emerges in the therapeutic field to give a sense of coherence to the chaos of emotions and sensations.[24] He pointed out that it is not a logical process and used the term *selected fact* to describe this emotional experience.[25] He clarified that it is the result of the analyst's ability and the emotional experience of working together as a group or couple. In *Transformations*,[26] Bion added that when he thought he grasped his patient's meaning, it was often "by virtue of an aesthetic (italics in original) rather than a scientific experience". So, if we consider these features of the process, it could be postulated that in mother-child therapy the baby might have an active role in the emergence of an aesthetic selected fact.

The second tool is the possible use of "imaginative thinking".[27] The most archaic memory traces, including those about earliest traumas, can be registered only in non-representational form. In *Taming Wild Thoughts*,[28] Bion again wrote that in his opinion, in addition to conscious and unconscious states of mind, there may be another one, which he referred to as "inaccessible". It manifests itself through somatic innervations and is expressed physically through basic emotions experienced as excessive. In this work, Bion again highlights the importance of *aesthetic* elements, in both the sensory and artistic meaning of the word, on the road towards formulating scientific sentences in an analytic context.[29] So in my clinical experience, I attempted to gather up the baby's and mother's sensations as a first step towards sensory integration, a first "common relational sense shared relational meaning" a "first sense of truth" in each subject and between them. The vitality of beta elements in the baby and their urge to evolve towards sensory integration can be used as a bridge to help the mother's defensive sensory disintegration. Later this first integration will be able to evolve into a "truth-functional-statement", a second level of mental functioning, a more verbal representative one.

Clinical case

Through many years of analysis, Valentina was a young woman who had tried to extricate herself from a borderline psychic[30] situation and severe food disturbance. Following the birth of her daughter, she had another breakdown, and in the wake of an incident that endangered her baby, she decided to begin a new therapy. We started mother-baby therapy. The session reported here occurred four months after we had begun. The baby, Anna, was eight months old. We sat together on the carpet.

Valentina: I went to see the paediatrician who scolded me about Anna's poor diet. Many foods are bad for her, like cheese, vegetables, and flour. I tried giving her some milk at supper, but she refused it and wanted to eat our food.

I feel scared as the paediatrician. I think I rushed into the movie *Hungry Hearts*, where a traumatised mother tries to manage her anguishes by controlling the baby's food to severely malnourished and death risk. I also think this mother experiences any transformation with anguish and says so in concrete ways. So, as not to be experienced the transference as the paediatrician, I feel the need to consider that she shares dependence as a form of persecution. I know that Valentina can't access a knowledge level, but I don't know how to empathise with her difficulties without feeling myself a potential killer of the baby.

Analyst: When we aren't sure what's good and evil, we have to go by trial and error.
Valentina: The paediatrician didn't talk down to me. She was even kind, but in her opinion, vegetables don't give you constipation. That's not how I see it.

It seems that Valentina renounces to engage a fight with me. I also think there seems to be a hint of a healthy element in the way she prioritises the relationship with her baby. I wonder if I am trying to find something good in a dangerous situation only to prevent being overwhelmed by fear.

Valentina tried to contain herself, but a "catastrophic emotional explosion"[31] was in the field. I try to give her back the capacity to feel competent about her baby's needs, but my words cannot sound emotionally true.

As we speak, baby Anna takes hold of the tail of a rat toy and explores it, all the while checking surreptitiously for her mother's attention, stopping and starting many times. Anna carefully explores the objects around her and displays the features of curiosity and inhibition linked to the many traumatic situations experienced during her life. We are speaking about what her mother considers dangerous food, and now, exploring the toy rat with her mouth, I imagine she takes a small step from reality to play. Anna leads us to contemplate and explore unpleasant and even disgusting things. Finally, she does something to contain herself searching for the mother's help.

As in a therapy group, I decided to mirror the possible progression process.

Analyst: [in an ironic tone of voice and looking at the mother first and then the baby] We speak about dangerous food, and Anna is tasting a rat. That's quite a brave step!

Valentina seems not to consider my words but surprising me, the concreteness of dangerous foods becomes a telling of a harmful interaction.

Valentina: Last night, I had trouble getting Anna to sleep again. I got wound up, and after a while, I burst into tears and wanted to go away. My husband arrived and tried to help me, but I hated him because he thought I was a bad mother, and at the same time, I wished I could make Anna quieten down concretely. [She starts crying.]

There are strange, consensual movements of mother and baby in an area that somehow resembles a transitional space between the body and mind, the effort to contain bad feelings and evacuate them. Valentina tells about her need for mental food in the relationship and her inability to take it inside. Again, I feel myself worried about the possibility of new actions, and, at the same time, I find myself considering the baby as a subject in the field able to start a new transformation.

Anna explores the soft toy and seems fascinated by the labels coming out from its seams.

The labels belong to the object but are at the same time something different and outside of it.

It seems that the baby is engaged in an unconscious dialogue with her mother. While the mother explores her feelings, the baby parallels transformations with her body, using her mouth and fingers to scan the object and discover something connected to it but a bit different.

Analyst: I knew a grandmother who made a toy for her grandchildren by sewing different labels onto a ribbon.

There is no reflexive thinking in these words, but, in *après-coup*, it is possible to consider them as an attempt to create a picture of the process. In the grandmother character, it is possible to include all the subjects in the relational field who are trying to sew different mind levels.

Valentina: Wash and iron care labels?
Analyst: Yes. [after a quiet pause] I've just had a strange fantasy: I imagined Anna waving her arms around last night and conjuring up a label with 30% tiredness and 70% fear written on it.

Anna starts to whine as if experiencing our ability to help her after the transformative psychic work. Valentina picks up her baby rather roughly and says:

Valentina: Yesterday night, I think that I washed Anna with rather hot water!

Valentina shows how her body and mind are both experiencing difficulties in transforming pain. Last night was painful, but so is the memory of her act of violence just after the baby's birth. I feel that in her rude gesture to pick up her baby, Valentina also shows something of her childhood experience. At six years of age, Valentina's mother lost her brother, four years old, invested by a motorcycle while he was on her attention. So this woman couldn't take care of Valentina without transmitting the gestures of taking care, the unbearable agony of the fault. So, I attempt to put these thoughts into words.

Analyst: You know how it is when we think a dress is finally spotless, but then we look at it in the sunlight only to discover that the stain is still there. I felt that perhaps Anna sometimes makes you feel not good enough, and this feeling is like a stain within yourself. I think that your mother felt the same as you.

Valentina is thinking, and, probably to get her mother's attention, Anna lets her body slide down from her mother's arms; this movement puts Valentina in another difficult situation as she tries to contain her baby both in body and in mind. Now, the mother has to govern oscillations from mind to body containment. Valentina is upset about her capacity to cope. The baby's body reflects the situation of the mind-body disconnection linked to the trauma of the grandmother. Her mother's unconscious anxiety and fault damaged her ability to use her mental container. The ontological anxiety overwhelmed the balance between body and mind, and complex defenses tried to protect the mind by using the body to evacuate.

It came to my mind the paintings of German artist George Baselitz, who became famous for his ability to paint his subjects upside down; this memory enables me to reconnect with my imaginative thinking and use the reverie to sustain the dreaming capacity of the mother. To do that, I feel I had to use the body, not the words.

Analyst: Anna is in the same position as during birth, and you are in the same pain.

I try to make myself a midwife to help the mother contain and transform the emotions and sensations in the field, starting from the body: taking the baby's head in my hands, I help them search for each other, saying little sentences, describing feelings and movements. At first, Anna encounters her mother's scared expression and starts to cry. Then she explores the mother's face with her mouth and fingers and seems fascinated by her mother's hair as by the labels on the toy. Finally, she trusts enough to connect herself to the object.

Three years later

I want to show that the child can help the mother face the oscillation between primitive feeling and representation, body and mind in another development point. Valentina had improved her capacity to take care of her daughter, but sometimes her primitive anguishes slip again into the body of her child. When the child was three years old, there were constipation moments, as happens typically in development. These transitory moments communicate through the body the child's usual fear of losing pieces of herself and the desire for control over the losses imposed by progressive greater separation from the mother. Valentina lived these moments as dangerous for the child and a sort of entrapment for herself. Again, with the unconscious intention to wash away negative feelings, she administered massive doses of laxative to the child. But, again, not being able to perceive herself as a separate subject, she projected her difficulties into the child; after acting, she feels herself exposed to crises of the anguish of having damaged her child to the point of causing her death. Moreover, Anna began to attend kindergarten confronting her mother with further difficulty in separation. Valentina told me in the session that she found herself trapped in a nightmare from which she couldn't wake up. Again separation became inside Valentina a fear of death; the unrepresented feelings of her mother arose inside her, and the only solution was to project them inside the body of her child. We often speak about constipation, trying to connect the concrete situation to the entrapment in which her feelings jailed her, but with no result. For example, Valentina gives her daughter some laxatives every day to prevent constipation, causing diarrhea. The body symptom pushes Valentina to feel guilty for damaging her child, but only two days of no evacuation make her mad again.

One day in a session without the baby, who remained at home for flu, Valentina asked to show me two videotapes on her phone: first, she and Anna were singing a particular song from the Disney film *Frozen*, and in the second, we can see Anna waking up. Valentina wants to show me her capacity to confront this difficult moment. I thought about how waking up for Valentina meant a need to freeze her unrepresented feelings and project them into her daughter's body, along with the hope of a new opportunity at a later date for unfreezing, re-experiencing and correcting the original maternal failure situation. Winnicott indicated as in treatment "a new and reliable environmental adaptation [which] can be used by the patient in correction of the original adaptive failure [of the early maternal environment]."[32] I hypothesise that it could be facilitated by experience to be in treatment together with her baby.

Valentina was describing to me how the anguish persecutes her all over the day, starting from when she had to go out to work, and at the same time, she wanted to share her new capacities in taking care of Anna. While she was talking, she remembered a drawing of her daughter that she had taken in her bag. It was a squiggle with a little inside line of different colors.

Valentina explained to me that one morning Anna told her she was as afraid of going to kindergarten as she was of going into a dark cave (the squiggle represented the cave). Valentina said to the child that in the dark cave lived little people (the colored lines drown by the child): she drew the sun and the rays like lines entering the cave up to the single little character. This drawing and the storytelling of the mother served the function of helping the baby stop crying and accept to go to kindergartner.

The child starts to represent her fear, and the mother does the same; she can understand through this primitive sign something about her going down in the dark more than with my words. Like in Winnicott's squiggle play, the active participation of both subjects effectively transforms the unconscious feelings of both.

Analyst: Anna represented the kindergarten as a cave, and you transformed it into a light-full place inhabited by colorful characters. You conserved the drawing as a precious object in your bag, and for this, we can hypothesise it represents something more than a simple drawing. It contains something of your experience too.

Valentina: The drawing let me feel active and effective, in contact and different from Anna at the same time.

Analyst: Two bodies in contact and two minds in oneness. You have been brilliant in catching Anna's effort to communicate her fear.

Valentina: The problem sometimes isn't Anna's fear but my terror of losing her. It is like a dark ink that erases my mind.

Analyst: You fall into a dark cave that makes you feel blind and prisoned. But now Anna can start to make her presence, and you, like a bat, have a radar to find her.

I thought that the squiggle could be seen from a different point of view and represent a crucial moment in the process. It represents a first attempt of Anna to share her little capacity to contain feelings and the dark hole in which she goes down when her mother becomes unable to help her. Valentina finds in the squiggle a mirror of her experience. The pre-representational form is more able to enter her mind and be assimilated without directly using the primitive defences to wash away the negative.

The baby as the effective probe to explore the analytical field

The "open field" is, from a psychoanalytic point of view, a helpful device for observational purposes and for the exploration of new ways of expanding knowledge and improving therapeutic outcomes.

Using Bion's grid, the open field is like a periodic table that enables us to observe transformations in different directions whilst also trying to reverse development and use the concept of oscillation more freely.

Bion described how the mother could use her reverie to transform the baby's body communication into pictograms and meaning. However, her task is to transform the meaning into a gesture to give back its sense to the baby. Starting from this description, Bion revealed further developments in his theory, a first description of the oscillation between body and mind, gesture and thinking and the interweaving of the two subjects of the relationship.

Let us suppose that a mother is experiencing the inability to be an adequate container, starting with her body. As a result, the beta elements inside her and the elements evacuated by the baby will remain untransformed, and she will be unable to help her infant with her mind or body. It happened when the mother was a victim of trauma in the early stage of development. She had to freeze her catastrophic feelings and hide them on an unconscious, deep level that is not accessible by memory. When she does experience taking care of the baby, she is pushed in her experience, in the place of breakdown.

Without the mother's help, the baby cannot process his raw emotional experiences, evacuate them, and thus fails to develop the capacity to learn from experience.

In the preceding clinical experiment, at the beginning of therapy, Valentina expressed difficulty in containing and processing her negative emotions by projecting them onto food for her child. Food thus became potentially harmful, and the only way to protect the child was to deprive her of food.

I described how the analyst could help the oscillation between baby and mother containment by using the baby's body to reactivate the mother's capacity to offer containment first through her body. The baby was developing its container, and the initial stage (proto-container) intersected with the broken development of the mother.

Using the permeability of the physiological regulation between infant and mother, I hypothesised that the baby wasn't only a container of projected negative emotions but might select something pertinent and potentially valuable for the relational situation.

With due consideration of the baby's fragility, I attempted to use the selected fact emerging in the field to foster emotional contact between mother and baby; being unable to achieve a relationship with the body traps the patient in unthinkable anxiety that can drive her to madness and death. The analyst's role is to facilitate the transformation of the raw and unmodulated feelings from the body in an internal musical dimension starting from aesthetic elements. The analyst may follow the tracks of bodily communication and the physical connection to revitalise the mind's transformative function. We can also consider what happens between the subjects involved in a psychoanalytical relationship as the field theory perspective allows, better than other theories. What we can observe is always the result of a conscious and unconscious interaction in which it is impossible to decide the weight of contribution of each subject. From this point of view, the baby may be considered a sensitive probe able to explore the dynamic field and capture relevant issues to start a transformation. For the same reason, the analyst's interpretation could describe the emerging link between unconscious feeling more than the unconscious meaning emerging in one of the subjects. Moreover, the more unsaturated baby's communications increase imagination and daydreaming.

Judith Herman,[33] whose *Trauma and Recovery* is still a classic text, states that the reestablishment of a safe space is the first step in recovery. Safety is a place of containment, as well as a person who can listen without being overwhelmed. In such a space that therapy represents, the surprising emergence of considering the baby, the weakest subject, as the more effective one to transform body sensations into mental ones needs more exploring but could be an effective research field to help mothers with complex mental difficulties.

Notes

1 Ferro 2006; Ferro and Basile 2009; Ferro and Civitarese 2015.
2 Grotstein 2007; Marks-Tarlow 2015.
3 Bion 1963, p. 22.
4 Ogden 2004.
5 Ferro 2009.
6 Grotstein 2007.
7 Cartwright 2016.
8 Bion 1962a, p. 306.
9 Bion 1975, p. 148.
10 Cartwright 2010.
11 Lombardi 2017.
12 Bion 1975, p. 67.
13 Bion 1975, p. 67.
14 "With psychotic patients, the bodily sensations are sometimes the only way to create a 'place in which [the patient] could feel that he exists'" (Ogden 1989, p. 130).
15 Mawson 2019; McKinley et al. 2012.
16 Bion 1997b.
17 Winnicott 1974, p. 88.
18 Bion 1970.
19 Levine et al. 2013; Scarfone 2015.
20 Bion 1967b, 1970; Winnicott 1971c, p. 94.
21 Salomonsson 2014.
22 Fraiberg 1975.
23 Reiner 2010.
24 Bion 1962b.
25 The expression "selected fact" was borrowed by Wilfred R. Bion from the French mathematician Henri Poincaré who referred to this concept as the element that makes it possible to give coherence to a group of scattered data.
26 Bion 1965, p. 52.
27 Bion 1997b, pp. 6–7.
28 Bion 1997b, p. 50.
29 Salomonsson 2006; Civitarese 2013.
30 All names and other identifying information have been changed to protect patient identity.
31 Bion 1970.
32 Winnicot 1954, p. 293.
33 Herman 1997.

Chapter 2

Intimacy and autism

An apparent paradox

Is it possible for a therapist to become "autistic" when working with an autistic person? The question is deliberately ambiguous and provocative.

The concept of emotional intimacy involves the idea of being open to others and on the same wavelength; on the other hand, patients with *Autistic Spectrum Disorders* (ASDs) have a hard time dealing with relationships. For this reason, becoming "autistic" for a therapist is an emotional paradox: becoming autistic means seeking empathy with the patient, but also sometimes protecting the self, unconsciously, from contact with overwhelming feelings. Maintaining the paradox can be a valuable tool in psychoanalytic therapy.

ASDs refer to a range of neurodevelopmental disorders that include autism itself and related conditions. Many possible etiological factors are recognised, including genetic and environmental ones, but psychogenic factors have progressively been seen as less important. So psychoanalytic treatment, which puts these at the core of therapy, gradually lost importance, to the point that for many years psychoanalysis was viewed as a low-efficacy treatment.

Psychoanalysts know and share beliefs with neurological and behavioral specialists about many of the factors, but they have a certain specificity in their way of elaborating theoretical models to explore the processes involved in transforming emotions. Moreover, in the scientific world, there is a new consideration that interventions should not be limited to the external adjustment of maladaptive behaviors while ignoring the internal experience – the emotions, fantasies, and anxieties. Effective interventions should aim at activating, "from within," the individual's interactive, intersubjective, reciprocal, and emotional sharing skills. The difficulty these patients have of perceiving time and space as normotypical people, as well as their inability to perceive the other as a whole subject, prevents most of them from using language, the main tool to fill the void in which they feel immersed.[1]

This chapter therefore aims to examine what it means for the analyst to become autistic in the therapeutic process, to explore, together with the patient, intimate psychic relationships and to build a possible shared sense of space and time starting from the body's perceptions.

DOI: 10.4324/9781003388838-3

Within the complexity of the analytical process, three aspects in particular will be considered:

1 specificity in bodily contact
2 different ways to build meaning
3 the possibility of interpretation through body performance.

Caravaggio and his painting *Boy Bitten by a Lizard*

An aesthetic example can help to imagine different ways of processing pain, which are sometimes revealed through a form of bodily communication.

In his painting *Boy Bitten by a Lizard*, Caravaggio depicts a young man whose face is deformed by pain. The effect is increased by the asymmetry of the face, and this distortion is probably due to the optic lens used by the artist as a drawing aid.[2]

The face in particular is the result of two different painting moments: one in which the boy is depicted more frontally, and a second in which he is shown more laterally (see Figure 2.1). Indeed, the use of an optic lens obligated the painter to create the painting by dividing it into parts and then reassembling these.

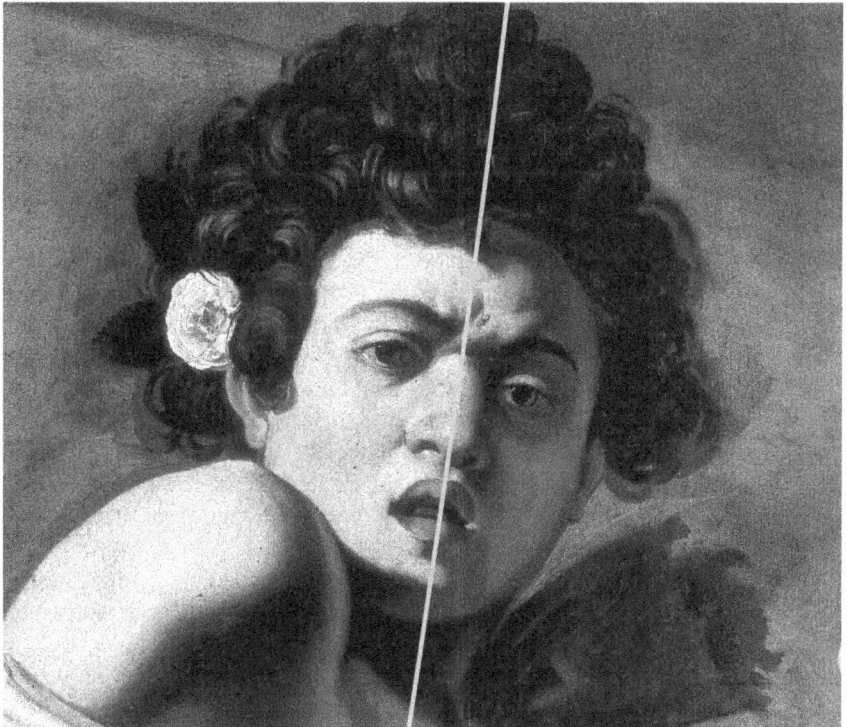

Figure 2.1 Caravaggio's *Boy Bitten by a Lizard*.

This painting is useful in illustrating how a neurotypical and an autistic person can bodily communicate pain from two different points of view. Nonverbal communication, especially when expressed in the face, is a common way to transmit emotions; however, autistic children don't decode the emotional features of the face, relying instead on clues manifested in other parts of the body and on repetition.

Caravaggio's depiction can also be used to visualise how an analyst might try to re-create in his mind the sudden pain that can penetrate the analytic relationship, like a lizard's bite, when the child patient enters a loop of repetitive gestures. It can be hypothesised that the beginning of the loop is a painful sensation that is difficult to comprehend or to transform into emotion. So the analyst needs to put together different ways of perceiving the situation, and then, like a painter using a lens, he can transform the different view into a mental image.

Before giving a clinical example of this type of transformation, in which the line that connects two ways of experiencing pain functions as an important locus of transformation, the following experiment explains how this technical tool can be developed.

Learning to see from another point of view

An artistic experiment, a sort of sensorial calligraphic experience similar to a Japanese one conducted by Steve Jobs, was the first step of changing the point of view of some of the relational features encountered with autistic children.[3,4] In particular, the tactile experience became the starting point for a new way to look at the autistic patients' productions.

In this artistic encounter, each participant was blindfolded and then told to put his hand into ten different bags containing unknown materials: little round stones, pieces of moss, broken tiles, feathers, and so on. With the other hand, each had to draw, on a square piece of cardboard, the transformation of this tactile experience into a graphic one. To facilitate a more accurate translation from a tactile sensation to a two-dimensional shape, the participants could choose to use either the rough or the smooth side of the cardboard, and they could also choose – without looking – either a pencil with hard or soft lead, a graphite stick, or a charcoal stick.

At the end of the experiment, after removing the blindfold, each participant could view the ten pieces of cardboard he had created, as a sort of tactile, visual, almost musical arrangement. Each piece was clearly different from the other but also deeply linked to each other by their sensorial origins.

Moreover, in each cardboard it is evident as without using sight, touching and hand movements push to return to a stage in which the imagination is not a symbolic imagination but a sensorial one.

Bringing this experience into the clinical office and observing, for example, the patient's repetitive gesture of touching an object or pushing a toy car back and forth, a new possibility to observe with tactile sense and not with sight could start.[5] Given that sight is closely connected to both relational and symbolic development, it becomes the dominant sense early in childhood. At the same time, it can form an obstacle to change the point of view with which the experiences with autistic children are processed.

The obstacle was evident also in the artistic experiment in the opportunity to confront and then to transform the difficult feeling of sight deprivation. The experiment took about an hour, and though at first curiosity and excitement for the new prevailed, as time went on, it was not easy to accept being in the dark. The dark arouses anxiety in the same way as an autistic child is forced to feel a primitive type of sensation and put aside the meaning that the sight immediately suggests. Another important feature of the experiment was the transformation of touching into a movement that can produce a sign but not a symbol. The movement of the hand in relation to cardboard squares became a way to explore them in their singularity and to discover as the objects can flow together to form a current of action. In everyday life, hand movements and expressive facial movements process and reveal inner experience in a sub-symbolic way. These movements are crucial features in positioning oneself in relation to one's surroundings. This system is also crucial in registering frame-by-frame movements and word-by-word conversations, allowing the subject to engage and accommodate the other's presence.[6]

The art experiment became the prototype for a similar one in the therapy room. Observing a child repeat the same gesture as though in a loop, the artistic experiment made it possible to imagine being blind and touching the gesture, trying to transform it into a "middle gesture" and to accept the terrifying feeling that initially arose in the field and in each of the subjects. The expression "middle gesture" suggests the process with which the analyst tries to reproduce a mixture of something of the patient's gesture with his own sensations and feelings utilising senses other than sight. Movement achieves something symbolic and not symbolic at the same time – something like a sign, not a word or a drawing. At the same time, gesture isn't a simple mirror of the child's; in the analyst's mind, the movement blends sensation and an initial attempt at transformation. So the analyst makes himself into the line extending between the patient's sensorial word and his need to transform it into a meaningful fact. Usually therapists are trying to look at repetitive actions, drawings, and movements as potentially meaningful situations; this is an important feature in mental development, but sometimes an autistic child can feel this process too unfamiliar and respond by strengthening his defenses.

Using the tool called the "middle gesture" reduces the time before the patient emerges from repetition and pushes the autistic patient to find with the analyst a more symbolic way to communicate. Something more about the "middle gesture" can be explained by drawing from the performing arts, and in particular, by Marina Abramovic's performances.

The performance: a way to integrate gesture and emotions

Performance is a form of art that implies the active involvement of an audience, and the relationship with audience members is not established by the object itself but by the performing artist's body. The performing artist does not know the outcome of the interaction, as it is open to the unpredictable contribution of the audience. In the performing arts, the body conveys emotions and meanings in an unstable balance between the creative intuition at the base of the piece and the unpredictable response of the audience that makes the artwork concrete. The performance artist therefore has a very special relationship with the audience and needs to practice surrendering in the presence of the other, integrating the other into the mind and actions without being overwhelmed.[7] The performance does not aim to close the gap between artist and audience through an object loaded with meaning, but rather it opens up the possibility of maintaining a space where the contributions of spectators create a link that extends across that space. In calling on the public to participate, the performer proposes an aesthetic experience and a transformational process. So, in a work of performance art, the distance between the actor and the people experiencing the performance is different from that in all other artistic situations; like a mother who has just given birth, the artist is not an object but a transformational process.[8] The "aesthetic moment" of performance, as Bollas[9] called it, can put the subject in contact with deep sensations, memory, and feeling, achieving no discourse other than presentational symbols.[10]

Performance artist Marina Abramovic, in particular, used her body to achieve different steps in the process of studying interactions between artist and audience. In the first cycle of performances, she used her body to transform the pain and vulnerability experienced in her childhood, re-creating a masochistic situation – that of trying to attract the attentive gaze she never received from her mother.

During a second period, Abramovic produced performances in partnership with her boyfriend, Ulay. This time the pivotal point was to experience trust, intimacy and commitment, along with the relationship between the bodies of the artists and the public. In a third period, Abramovic became an artist who valued the performance field as a space for transformative experiences, including experiences without movement. In her performance called *The Artist Is Present*, she remained silent and motionless for many hours a day; on the rare occasions when she met the eyes of people sitting in front of her, there were intense emotional reactions. Only by shutting and then reopening her eyes when a spectator before her was having such a reaction could she create a situation of deep intimacy.

These performances allow for links with the therapeutic process of autistic children. Tustin suggested that, if autism is a wordless illness, it must be treated without words; thoughts and emotions (etymologically, something that "moves outward") come from bodily sensations, and their transformation may be better expressed through action.[11,12] Abramovic's performances allowed something else useful for therapy to be grasped.

Tustin[13] described autism as a "sensation-dominated state in which perception is elementary, restricted, or grossly abnormal"; she qualified it as "perverse self-sensuality". Tustin's word *perverse* does not refer to sexual behaviors, of course, but rather, from a certain point of view, it captures something present in the relational field when a repetitive gesture or other apparently unmeaning action pervades the relationship between the analyst and the autistic child. To trust and enter into mental intimacy with the patient, the therapist must undergo a sort of submissive process in order to see as the patient sees. In a therapeutic relationship with an autistic child, this process has the features of a "doer and done-to" relationship – a sadomasochistic way of being together. Feeling trapped, as many authors have described, is a common experience for the analyst treating autistic children. The risk of this feeling is that the analyst may attempt to protect himself by employing tough defenses that are not so different from autistic ones. Conversely, working through the feeling of being bullied and transforming it into an attitude of trusting surrender is the first step in the transformative process.[14,15,16]

The first time of Abramovic's performances, sleeping into masochistic features, allows one to intuit that a particular gesture can be simultaneously a defense against pain and also part of a transformative process. In the beginning, spectators responded to Abramovic's masochistic passivity as a sadistic group, as in a Bionian basic assumption, but the same group was gradually able to exit this role and allow a transformation of the artist, too. In therapy, the role of suffering pain and eventually of escaping from the trap of "doer and done to" rests with the analyst, but paradoxically, it becomes possible only with the participation of the patient, as in Abramovic's performances.

In some ways, the first clinical vignette presented has things in common with this type of performance, as I try to show.

Touching and smelling as a dangerous situation

Charles is a child with an ASD of medium severity. He was adopted when he was three months old, after having been abandoned. He started psychotherapy at age three years, about one year following the first appearance of autistic symptoms. In addition to psychotherapy, he participated in a program for language development and made regular visits to a public health center where his neuropsychiatric progress was evaluated.

Charles's mother decided to include private psychotherapy in her son's care program because she thought that his very early abandonment may have played a role in the etiology of the disease. Though this cannot be scientifically validated, she was a very sensitive mother who had experienced psychotherapy herself, and she wanted her child to have the same opportunity to encounter and explore feelings. She said: "He comes from abroad, and I want him to be able to find his country of origin hidden in his body." This very touching sentence referred not only to her child's Asian facial features but also to his biological mother and to all that was hidden, not understood in their relationship. Probably, Charles's adoptive mother also needed help herself in coping with painful aspects of the adoption process, as well as with Charles's unexpected problem.

I have been working with Charles two times a week and with his parents once a month. I will relate two vignettes that occurred when he was five years old.

During a summer session, I was wearing sandals. Charles looked down at my painted toenails and, lying down on the carpet, he started to smell my feet. I was embarrassed and tried to calm myself by thinking about how animals construct odor maps to recognise certain sites, just as newborn humans do. Charles proceeded to touch my feet, wanting to pull off my sandals, and even though I tried to stop him, he put his face onto my feet, exploring them with his mouth. He looked very excited, and it was difficult for me to accept this violation of normal social rules governing body intimacy. I found myself wondering up to what point I had to allow Charles to lick my feet, to submit to something that was for me not exciting at all and in fact rather unpleasant. I was in a relationship in which I felt something was perverting my feeling, pushing me to pass from trust to defense. On the other side, a part of me needed to transform this experience preserving relationship as if I had to pass, inside my mind, from Abramovic's first period performances to the second ones.

I remembered a 1977 performance by Abramovic and her boyfriend, Ulay: the couple stood naked on either side of the entrance to the Galleria d'Arte Moderna (Community Gallery of Modern Art) in Bologna, Italy. The narrowness of the space forced visitors to squeeze sideways between them, compelled to choose between facing either the naked Ulay or the naked Abramovic. The public was confronted with the embarrassing position of visual and physical contact with the performers.

As in that performance, I had to go forward with Charles and enter into a symbolic place (the art museum), but first I had to pass between two naked bodies: my feet and the child who was smelling and licking them, together representing a very tight door.[17] I tried to blank my mind to social embarrassment, finding intrigue in something new; my feelings were close to those of a newborn having its first sensorial impressions of the world, attracted to the brightness of light and color and smells. I thought to myself that, for Charles, initial sensorial impressions might remain exciting but nothing more, lacking the start of a transformation process in which they could become something more, contributing to maturity in sign and form with meaning and relational limits.

Continuing to think of Abramovic's performance, I was able to submit to the wonder of the other and to force myself to take off my sandals. I then used red tempera paint to make imprints of my feet on a large sheet of paper, trying to enter into a symbolic space through the intermingling of bodily contacts. Taking inspiration from me, Charles started to make imprints with his hands, and then together we made squiggles with both our feet and hands, entering in this way into our very own art exposition.

A different way to process space and time

Relativity is an important theory with which to explore physical phenomena, but it is also a useful metaphor for describing the non-linear relationship between time, motion and space perception from a psychological point of view.[18] Perception isn't an exact picture of reality; time doesn't move in one direction, and in the human mind, time is a puzzle more intricate than a Newtonian scientist might expect. Temporal perception is an important factor in human emotions and mental health;

without awareness of time, it is not possible to imagine the future or to give order to the past.[19]

Conscious and unconscious precognition is a cognitive and affective way to prevent the mind from noticing unexpected facts. Experimental research has demonstrated that this process is important in priming reinforcement and memory, such that effects can operate backward in time.[20] Time and space share a great deal of geographical/biological overlap in the human brain, and experimental evidence shows that time and motion perceptions are linked, sharing common neural underpinnings.[21]

Psychotherapists observe spatiotemporal structure from a different point of view – as operational space-time based on neuronal, internal and exteroceptive stimuli, but in particular on relationships and emotions. From a psychological point of view, time and memory as characterised in clinical psychoanalytic accounts have a puzzling relationship; thus, the same memory can be referred to in a very different way at the beginning of therapy than at the end. Moreover, space and time in dreams are organised following a different schema than in conscious daytime life – or as Matte-Blanco[22] observed, they follow alternative logical hypotheses. Sometimes space and time in the therapeutic setting can be used without cognitive reference and simply as aesthetic narrative features with which to communicate emotions.[23]

Even if psychotherapists are familiar with this non-cognitive way of processing space and time, it is difficult to grasp an autistic way of functioning. Yet everyone is hard pressed to find the survival advantage offered by a solid grasp of a usual way of processing facts. Nevertheless, analysts in particular are attempting to discover something more in the functioning of the autistic mind. Child analysts, especially, are trained in deep-body communication and infant observation, and they are effective in catching the nuances of emotions expressed through the body.[24] While space is more connected to the biological experience of sight and movement, time is an abstract concept. Persons affected by ASD have problems with memory, but this may be only the most evident consequence of a different way of perceiving facts in the time-space frame. Not always do such patients experience the passing of time because they are concentrating on space as a sequence of scenes linked not by time but by other logic.[25,26]

The artistic experiment, referred to earlier, gave me occasion to change my mind about the sense of time and space and to view these in an autistic way to process the experience and their role in linking different actions. The starting point for my observation was the product of the artistic experience: ten little squares marked with different signs but linked by size, type of paper, and the experience of working through. I saw them as a sequence, similar to a musical score or the frames of film that form a movie (see Figure 2.2).

Another suggestion came from my memory of Abramovic's performance, *The Artist Is Present*. Here she remained static and silent, sitting on a chair for eight hours a day, allowing visitors to New York's Museum of Modern Art to spend a few minutes in the seat facing her. What I want to underline is a detail of this performance: Abramovic closed her eyes when a visitor got up to leave and opened them

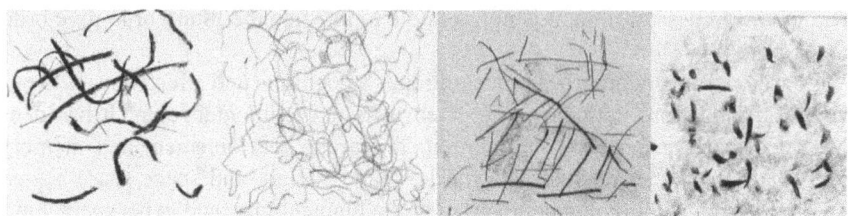

Figure 2.2 The sequence of tactile signs viewed as a musical score.

again when another person sat down in their place. This opening and closing of eyes was a symbolic movement in which Abramovic put forward the idea that looking might control spaces and other people, while simultaneously putting a limit on the artist herself and her capacity to contain her own and the other's feelings. The movement of opening and shutting the eyes decreased in some way the experience of a passing blur of unknown faces, reducing the effect of constant visual turnover on an internal domain.

After thinking about the art experience and this performance, I was more able to see how my patients' different actions were linked by the same shape and the same process of transforming different sensations. In a therapeutic situation with an autistic child, I began to look for the type of experience that the child was exploring, seeing it as broken into different actions. At the same time, I could reproduce within myself a feeling similar to Abramovic's in *The Artist Is Present*: that is, I paused to register the different actions passing by in the therapy room and tried to contain my own and Charles's emotions and to give meaning to the whole "performance".

Charles and the variable accuracy of a shape

In the following clinical vignette, I describe how Charles communicated something of his experience by locating the same anguished feeling in different situations.

Like many children with ASDs, the patient uses equivalency of body and mind, putting internal sensations outside; equivalency replaces identifications as a primitive method of relating. For an autistic child, I hypothesise that sometimes many different situations can be forcefully linked to one another not by something in the relationship – the meaning, the flow of emotions – but by the fluid shape of the edge between reality and its sensorial perception.[27,28] Sometimes a global experience can fill up the whole hour, even if it is pieced together from parts in which the child uses different senses and creates different sequences of motion. Often the use of a defensive shell arises around the exploration of dangerous edges, such as continuity-discontinuity, presence-absence or attraction-repulsion, and the child can spend the entire hour emerging from this terrifying feeling. Distinguishing when sensoriality is used in a defensive way from when it represents the first attempt to communicate – or, in other words, whether the patient is using a container or a proto-container – is a clinical problem that warrants further investigation.

During one session, Charles picked up a paper tube and started to make noises on it with sticks. He noticed that at the point where a tear in the tube was repaired with tape, the sound was different. He repeated this sequence many times. Then he drew a snail, and after many trials on different sheets of paper, he divided the spiral of the snail's shell into sections. He started to color his drawing, taking care not to color outside the lines; when this happened by accident, he stopped drawing and looked very distressed. He began to use his tongue to remove traces of color from his fingers, like a little cat. Then he pushed me to a place in the room where I was hidden behind a curtain, and if I attempted to come out, he would push me back again. He didn't look me in the eyes but used my body in such a way that it was clear he was not playing hide-and-seek.

When I told Charles that our time was almost up, he reacted by overturning a box of marbles. He wanted to pick up and return all the marbles to the box, sorting and aligning them and saying they were cookies. It was consequently very difficult to end the session. For the entire time, he had not reacted to my words or other types of interaction. Now he actively resisted ending the session. It gradually became evident to me that, during the session, I had tried to give meaning to different situations by capturing the emotions and using simple words to come as near as possible to describing the meaning of these different actions. I started to become able to shift from one sense to another (something like transmodal perception in a newborn), and I could see the different sequences fuse and link to each other in a way that I had not understood. I started to imagine that the link could take the shape of a global experience explored via different senses.

The first shape that I pictured in my mind to describe them was *continuity-discontinuity* – as manifested in sound (the tube), in three-dimensional space (the shell), on the skin (coloring that stuck to the fingers) and in the room (hide-and-seek). So I hypothesised that at the end of the session, separation was impossible to face not because of emotional pain but rather, the disturbing mix-up of marbles and the need to reorder them stood in for the emotional experience as a concrete, confusing situation.

Charles didn't want to stop. The next patient rang the bell. I went to open the door and then returned to the therapy room. I had two options: to force the patient to leave in haste, or to invent something that could describe the situation as it was taking shape in my mind and so to help him be ready to finish the session. In a few seconds, I realised that each sequence had been like a sensorial self-portrait that had no primary communicative intention, and that I could be in intimate communication with Charles through my body, performing the primitive meaning of continuity-discontinuity. Just as life and death are closely linked in the bodily experience of mother and child during labor and delivery, so the birth of meaning can be the same. To use my body to mirror my patient's experience, I had to essentially cancel the developing meaning and emotions inside me, instead coming into contact with much earlier, very primitive and rather disturbing sensations. There was a tension between abandonment and control, I felt. So I set myself in motion aimed at Charles, through the objects at hand, and I made the same gestures with the tube, the pencil, my tongue and so on, to represent mirroring. I felt desperate, as though

I were buried by these objects. Then I lay down on the floor (like a baby or a dead person), took all the objects and put them on top of me, I got up and let the objects fall down in disorderly fashion. Then I said to him: "It is the end. All are going away, but it isn't easy; it's like going down into a big confusion, just as happened with the marbles."

Charles then said, "Okay," and rather quickly accepted the ending of the session. When I was able to reflect, I thought that I had tried to communicate to Charles how I found it possible to understand the huge distance between us and between be and not to be. In some way, I wanted to show Charles that I had grasped the difficulty buried beneath his various actions; the end of the session confronted him not with the psychic pain of separation but with the interruption of his attempt to control falling down into a black hole of confusion.

Reaching the patient where he needs to be reached

Analytic proximity or intimacy with an autistic child includes the capacity to experience and give meaning to primitive states of being and emotions.

Autistic children defend themselves against primitive anxieties by using mimicry, psychic equivalency, suspension and dismantling; these defences create not only a distance between action and meaning but also a collapse of the vital body-mind unit and intimate relationship with the other.

The hypothesis was that what is observed, from a phenomenological point of view, is the result of a lack of integration of different levels of functioning and in particular of the containing function. This hypothesis was the first step toward considering the symptoms as a whole and abandoning the effort to find sense in each of them. But the prevalent containment function in an autistic child isn't mental but auto-sensuous. This patient use senses in a way that abolishes the distance between the self and the objects, an archaic way to be in contact with the other, but only through the body. The other, when perceived as a different subject, produces fear and sometimes terror.

In the analyst, this autistic defense produces a sense of impasse – a feeling of being kept out but sometimes also an unconscious closeness with the patient. In some ways, analyst and patient are both entering the same emotional withdrawal from the relationship.

When the analyst must reach the patient at the point where he is, it is not so easy to find a way to bridge the different ways of processing the experience. Starting with the premise that the body is not simply the unthinking portion of the mind-body system, the analyst can place the body and all relevant actions along a line of fragmentation, trying to build a bridge by drawing on the bodily participation of the child and the meaningful use of her own body.

The "middle gesture", like almost an artistic performance, arises only with the participation of the patient; it creates a primitive form of bodily communication. In some way, the renunciation of words depends on trust in the communicative power of the body. Abramovic's early performances helped to understand how a gesture can be considered as the intersection of many factors; it expresses the analyst's pain at being cut off, the overcoming of this pain, and the display of these feelings through the body – a way to share with the patient the same bodily level of expression. If these factors work together, the patient may feel that she has been reached and that the gesture can be shared.

Observing this hypothesis in action, a second one has arisen: in the autistic child, different sequences of action can be linked by the effort to confront the same fearful sensation. To discover it, the analyst has to concentrate more on the shape of the actions than on a single sequence, using a different logic that is closer to an artistic way of expressing emotion, drawing more on formal elements than on language. Using the "middle gesture", as a performance artist does, affords the possibility of building a shape of meaning that becomes alive only with the patient's participation.

The patient's response is then visible in a new form of intimacy, a transitional intimacy between body and mind. Through this therapeutic method, it may summarise the complex process of working through the transformation of impasse.

Thus, the autistic analyst's withdrawal from the relationship with patient, transformed into an experience near the body and sensoriality, became not only possible but helpful.

Notes

1 Amir 2014.
2 Hockney 2001; Landi 2000.
3 Isaacson 2011.
4 Steve Jobs related that a Japanese calligraphy course he took after leaving a more traditional university curriculum eventually became the starting point for the creation of the smartphone's touch screen. Touchable icons provided a more intuitive and faster way of interacting with the logic and complexity of computer functioning.
5 All the senses, including vision, are extensions of the tactile sense; the senses are a specialisation of skin tissue, and all sensory experiences are thus related to tactility. Our contact with the world takes place at the border of the self through a specialized part of our developing membrane (Pallasma 2005, pp. 10–11).
6 Bucci 1985, 1997.
7 Danckwardt and Wegner 2007.
8 Giannachi et al. 2012; Simões and Passos 2018.
9 Bollas 2015.
10 Langer 1953.
11 Tustin 1994b, p. 121.
12 Houzel (1997) writes that when he was in supervision with Tustin, he had the impression she was "thinking with her whole body'" (p. 344). After listening to what others said, she moved her hands, arms and body before talking, as if thinking arose not from the head but in the body.
13 Tustin 1972, p. 107.
14 Benjamin 2004.
15 Tustin 1994a; Durban 2014; Ahumada and Ahumada 2017.
16 Williams 1999; Molinari 2014; Korbivcher 2005.
17 Demaria 2004.

18 Appelbaum 2012.
19 Bem 2011; Bem et al. 2016.
20 Bem 2011; Bem et al. 2016.
21 Saj et al. 2014; Mauk and Buonomano 2004.
22 Matte-Blanco 1988.
23 Fonseca 2006; Molinari 2016.
24 How mentalisation is linked to language, and what role this plays in autism, is currently one of the most important fields of research on autism and language. Some recent research results (Fogassi 2007; Glenberg and Gallese 2012) suggest that imitation of movement, and not only sound imitation, can play an important role in learning language. Observing the use of space-time categories within the therapeutic relationship with an autistic child can shine a ray of light on the birth of language as well.
25 Rhode 2011.
26 Bick 1968; Alvarez 1999; Ahumada and Ahumada 2005, 2017.
27 Tustin 1987; Mitrani 1998; Lombardi 2008.
28 Alvarez 2010.

Chapter 3

One child, two parents, a psychoanalyst

In other words – a group

In Draft M to Fliess on May 25, 1897, Freud, after having abandoned the seduction hypothesis as the origin of neuroses, proposes to his friend the associative process of traumatic experience as he is portraying it at that point in his reflections. Contained in this text are important intuitions regarding the trans-generational, such as that the symptoms of sons and daughters are often replays and interpretations of the conflicts belonging to their parents or to other relatives who came before them.[1] Each member of a family has internal representations of the other members that are a composition of what he or she experiences in the present and, for parents, what they have experienced with their own families of origin. Such representations are therefore interwoven out of hidden feelings and desires, fantasies, stories and illusions that initially are not shared. It is against this intricate background of different stories, which Freud (1909) called the *family romance*, that the parents' request for help for their children takes shape. Indeed, it happens not infrequently that the family entrusts to the child, through a symptom, the role of spokesperson of conflictual dynamics, or they establish with the child a way of relating that itself becomes an intersubjective location of the little group of family members' unconscious.[2]

At the present time, an awareness that the child is part of a relational and fantasmatic system has led all child analysts, though belonging to different schools of thought, to agree on the necessity of establishing a therapeutic alliance with the parents. Over time various techniques for involving the family have been developed, moving from occasional meetings with parents as an adjunct to individual therapy with the child, to participatory sessions with one or both parents, to treatment of the family as a whole.[3]

Whichever setting is considered most appropriate for each situation, the child analyst must acquire the capacity to oscillate between individual therapy with the child and group therapy with the family, coming to a way of observing that Bion[4] defines as *binocular vision*. This arrangement allows for confrontation of the upset and its possible focalisation in the family's treatment, in which each of the subjects is exposed to a catastrophic experience of transformation that contains, anticipates and catalyses what isn't yet there. I will call this type of upset *psychoanalytic seeing,* borrowing the term from astronomy.[5] In fact, if every analysis can be a play, the treatment of a family is an amplified play since the analyst finds him-/herself at

DOI: 10.4324/9781003388838-4

the cross-roads of "many forces which appear in the field under many disguises,"[6] as happens in group therapy.

The experience of these difficulties has often already occurred in the initial meetings with the parents, in which the analyst can make of the experience something that intervenes between the story of the child's ailment and the fact that the center of the problem lies elsewhere. The possibility of picking up a trace of this undercover experience, which by analogy with radio Bion calls *interference*,[7] can be the beginning of a chance to transform aspects not yet accessible to meaning – in an image, an intuition, a memory that allows an early focus in common through words. This early experience, in addition, gives evidence of how the problem that analyst and parents propose to analyse together and what is manifested in the child may not be something that belongs to the past but is still in existence in the moment in which it is brought to light for study.[8] Far from Freud's archaeological model in which it was possible to excavate in search of buried objects in a relatively calm situation, interference manifests as a phenomenon closer to that described by Winnicott[9] in *Fear of Breakdown*, in which what was in the past is again found in the present with the same incandescence.

Interference, then, at first a weak signal of group suffering, can be perceived if the analyst utilises binocular vision – that is, the possibility of listening both to the conscious mind and the unconscious, permitting the analyst's internal gaze to focus in an oscillating way on both the subject and the group. Paradoxically, the child's suffering, which seems to be the more accessible part of the family's malaise, can become one of the ways that the group unconsciously mobilises obstacles to oscillation among the various perspectives, with the aim of avoiding mental pain that is not yet bearable.[10] If the analyst's binocular vision manages to remove itself from this focus on the child's symptom, it is then possible for it to be transformed from an obstacle into a resource.

As the group's passive subject – that is, as the subject that hosts suffering – the child can actively contribute to promoting the transformation of all the subjects of the group through movement, play, and drawing. Moreover, the valorisation of the child as a key element in the process of meaning-making through his or her primary receptivity of bodily and aesthetic elements limits the analyst's perception as the repository subject of knowing, protecting the therapeutic relationship, at least in part, from the parents' normal ambivalence. Finally, it's necessary to add a brief introductory consideration of the various possibilities for considering and dealing with erotic aspects that can permeate the relational field.

Today, in comparison to the time when Freud described it for the first time, childhood sexuality is an accepted fact that can be thought and managed by the analyst with sufficient mastery; but if one considers the child as a member of the family group and undertakes an extended treatment with the whole family, it can happen that erotic elements at first confined to the child are also manifested in the parents – in forms that involve the therapist in an emotional realm of turbulence and distortion of the possibility of observation.[11]

The theoretical perspective of the relational field allows one not only to consider erotic aspects as a psychophysical manifestation of sexual desire but also to remain vigilant about the aim of involvement and of mental coupling that these aspects activate.[12] The presence of erotic elements, due to the high emotional temperature they generate, can push the analyst toward defensive enactments, or simply accentuate primitive feelings of love, hate or curiosity.[13]

The word *passion*[14] seems appropriate to describe the push toward coupling in a broader sense, both physical and mental. Passion is thus a function of the field connected to the possibility of utilising primitive feelings without violence. In this sense, it is connected to reverie, which is simultaneously an effect and a way of expressing love.[15]

One can hypothesise that when it is present, passion, which can include metabolised erotic elements, represents a connection that reinforces the capacity to understand one another and promotes transformation of beta elements (raw sensory data) into alpha elements (units of meaningful experience).

Self-portrait with crossed hands

The parents of Adele, age four years, ask for a consultation following an urgent request by the teachers at her preschool because their child compulsively masturbates. The parents have difficulty using the word *masturbation*; they relate that Adele has rubbed her genitals since the age of six months, using the narrow band of her high chair which is placed between her legs to keep her from slipping out, and later rocking on whatever supportive object stimulates her in that area. At about two years of age, she began to use her hands, and the parents had tried many strategies to make her stop – dissuasion, threats, punishment – but all without result.

The parents' story produces in me a cinematographic effect: imaginatively, I picture Adele drawing, playing, acting capriciously, and then the visual field shrinks to her small hands, which the parents obsessively monitor – as though I am seeing the special effects of a wide-angle lens alternating with a telephoto lens.[16,17]

In the second meeting, the parents start to shift between themselves the responsibility for some of their educational choices, creating a climate of light emotional tension. The father begins to bite his fingernails, at first furtively and then in an almost embarrassing way. His teeth seem to inspect each finger, tearing away the little cuticles at the edge of each nail; the fingers enter the oral cavity and then come out accompanied by a small sigh of satisfaction. I find that something unusual is happening, in the sense that rarely in the first few meetings do patients allow private gestures to emerge, free of inhibitions. Only at the end of the session – perhaps giving voice to some of my own nonverbal expressions of astonishment and discomfort – does the mother state explicitly that her husband's nail biting is a gesture that he cannot seem to control, and for some months Adele, too, has begun to imitate him.

We adults agree to continue meeting for a while before initiating a formal observation of Adele. In subsequent sessions, I learn that the mom works as a physical therapist in a different city from where they live, and on her return home, not only does she see to the domestic chores and the dinner, but she also looks after her husband's grandmother, a very elderly woman who lives with them. She presents a very detailed account of all this caregiving to unburden herself of the sense of guilt she harbors at not having much time to devote to Adele. So her hands take care of many persons; they are concretely occupied both with the pain that inhabits the bodies of her patients, and the needs of her family members. But it is as though this pain is something that has to do with her own stifled needs; the pain continues to stick to her fingers.

Without being totally aware of it, when I review the meetings with these parents in my mind, I think of some of the images of Egon Schiele,[18] in whose pictures the hands are a central element and often in the foreground. These are gnarled hands, entangled, not infrequently of disproportionate dimensions in relation to the body, and capable of expressing a deep pain more than other details – such as posture or facial expressions – are able to do. In many self-portraits, furthermore, Schiele depicts his own hand with the fingers artificially separated, almost as though he wants to express, in consonance with the cultural movements of the early 1900s and with Freud's revolutionary ideas, the non-solidarity or non-unity of the ego.

After some meetings during which, together, we question ourselves about Adele's need to re-create a pleasurable situation even in apparently calm moments, I mention a possible link between pleasure and pain:

Analyst: I don't know if you have happened to see this, but a painter of the early 1900s, Egon Schiele, mixed eroticism and pain in his paintings. For example, you yourselves have told me that sometimes Adele has difficulty waiting for dinner to be ready, even if she is watching an animated cartoon that she likes. In short, sometimes the things that we like and we don't like get mixed together, and it's possible that Adele uses her hand to try to make pleasure predominate. We see this more when she masturbates, while what she doesn't like stays hidden.

This simple reference to pain has the effect of breaking open a dam that has held back not so much Adele's pain but pain that has inhabited her parents' lives. The mom is familiar with Schiele and seizes the opportunity provided by this visual association of mine to tell about the similarity in appearance between one of the painter's models and a friend of hers, who died in a road accident at the age of twenty years. Her description, more than that of her friend/sister, seems to be that of an alter ego – because, even though eight years have passed, the pain of this loss is very alive, and the grieving process has not even begun. She cries as she recalls this and says that even now she is not capable of going to the cemetery. Hence, during the session, I again reflect on the rupture of the self portrayed in Schiele's paintings by the separated fingers.

The contorted bodies that this painter puts forward not only communicate his own pain, but also, according to a recent interpretation, they are a partial reproduction of the figures of hysterical women photographed by Salpetrier.[19] These women somatised a pain that was private, but it was also connected to their social situation of marginalisation and denial of access to being recognised as subjects in their own right.

I think of this mom as a carrier of personal pain but also divided within herself between the effort to be recognised as a mother and as a woman. She is often oppressed by the tasks of caregiving and by the wish to maintain her own job; she wants to have the same rights as her husband, even as she takes his place in caring for his elderly grandmother. After my comment about the burden of caring for elderly persons who are not self-sufficient, the woman adds that for years she has also been caring for her mother-in-law (her husband's stepmother), even before their marriage.

I ask how her husband came to lose his mother, and I am told of her terrible death in a bedroom fire when he was five years old. The account of the fire had the effect of transforming this big man seated beside me into a small child who was overflowing with guilt. Adele's mother tells me that, before going to sleep, her husband's mother had asked him to close the window to avoid allowing the curtain to be moved by a breeze that could bring it into contact with the heater. He had obeyed her, but then his father had reopened the window and gone out of the room, returning only when a blaze had erupted and there was no possibility of saving the wife. The father of Adele's dad remarried, and the dad grew up with this new mother whom Adele's mom describes as unaffectionate, along with a father who had become decisively violent – as in the worst of the Brothers Grimm folk-tales. For this man, a happy ending comes in with his meeting the companion to whom he has entrusted the care of his stepmother. Her hands allow him to preserve the image of himself as a good little boy, keeping him safe from expressing feelings of hatred or rage.

Notwithstanding the fact that husband and wife unconsciously use each other in order to keep intact the usefully defensive arrangements that guarantee a certain compactness of the self, they experience their marriage as essentially satisfying, and they even plan to have a second child. First, however, they would like to resolve Adele's problem, fearful of the fact that a little rival could accentuate her obsession. At any rate, Adele's hands – just as in a picture by Schiele – are in the foreground, and they allow a glimpse both of erotic desire (understood as a new birth and a better realisation of the self) and of a body-mind that is painfully deformed by suffering.

As the treating therapist, I ask myself what my own analytic hands must do or not do. I think that a clear direction may be implicit in the parents' request to transform the masturbation. Transported into the analytic field, the masturbation appears to me as Adele's attempt to transform by herself a mixture of beta elements, a lump that instead needs at least one other mind in order to be thought. Thus, there is a clear warning for me as well: I must not be seduced by the pleasure of a way of caregiving that is nourished – like masturbation – more by fantasies than by a true meeting. It is a call to remain alert, one that necessitates observing this family's difficulties from different points of view and capturing in the field the passionate elements that promote mental coupling.

I recognise that the many stories alluding to death that the parents have brought up, linking themselves to personal losses, can create a depressive vortex within which one loses sight of Eros, of the elements of beauty and pleasure that are indispensable for transformations to occur. The imaginative reference to Schiele seems to me to be a precious element to be preserved in my mind as something attached to an aesthetic and representative model of transformation.[20]

For now, Adele, the imagined new baby, and the parents themselves, so complementary to each other and clinging together, sketch out in my mind the picture of a young, middle-class family in a composition of love and death (or mortification of the self), as in Schiele's last painting.[21]

The houses: construction of side-by-side containers

After some sessions in which I observe Adele together with her parents, the anti-Covid regulations relegate us to meeting behind a screen. The verbal conversation continues principally with the mom and with Adele, who stays in the room, playing partly on her own and partly interacting with her mom and me. The dad, on the other hand, disappears temporarily from the therapy because of his work, connected to the health emergency, which takes him away from home for about two months. This distancing, and the consequent loss of a certain family structure, is echoed in the contents of sessions during this period.

The mom tells of having received a turtle as a gift but of being afraid that, in digging in the dirt, it might go into the neighbor's garden. There follows a lengthy account of the neighbor, who is a person with whom one feels uncomfortable, in contrast to the other neighbor, who is kind and affectionate with Adele. This fear suggests to Adele's mom that she shouldn't keep the turtle and should instead entrust its care to her own mother.

Together with Adele, I am shown pictures of their garden on a tablet, including the turtle, and then the tree in which they would like to build a treehouse for the little girl. Adele then builds a series of houses with Legos, which she juxtaposes on a little table to form a sort of city landscape. She assembles the Legos, breaks them apart, and puts them together again, sometimes in an orderly way and at other times more chaotically.

I think about how the present uncertainty nourishes the desire for a secure shelter, a sort of hard shell adhering to her body, but such a shell cannot be considered sufficient because it is undermined by the use of the split, which includes as a consequence the feeling of being persecuted. The treehouse is an attempt to construct another refuge, one for the child self who feels attacked by the fantasma of ferocious animals – to which, however, it is difficult to give shapes and words beyond their location near home.

I search for a possible meaning in what Adele is doing, as though she, beyond being the *porte-symptôme*[22] of the group, can also be seen as the subject capable of participating in the creation of symbolic transformations. This way she has of arranging houses, juxtaposing them and showing them off with pride to her mom and me, demonstrates the desire for a closeness made current by the absence of her dad, but it is also the representation of her wish and that of her parents for containment and nearness. I ask Adele to tell me who lives in the houses, if there are other children living there. Adele answers that there are other people, but now the houses are shut up and the people cannot be seen.

That the motif of the house is an important sign of her relationship with her body and with her mother is noteworthy. Underlying the hypothesis that the house is a privileged symbol from which to explore the primary relationship is the fact that in the symbolic development of the healthy child, the house rises up to overlap with the representation of the body and is almost always the first representation of something other than the self. In this sense, it could be considered a pictogram of the primary relationship, a memory repository of having been in unison, an experience that arouses the fantasy of being able to transcend the separating space necessary in order to draw, and the experience that allows containment of the anxiety that the child encounters when she begins to do so. The house is a graphic or plastic outline of the memory of having had a body and mind in common, but it expands and also graphically offers a space in which to work through early feelings of distance. Moreover, the house is the mental location that restores a feeling of belonging and of familial intersubjectivity, which provides a dwelling place for the desire for durable ties that guarantee continuation of the generations.[23]

The representation of Adele is like an oneiric image: a condensation of an individuation of the family's subjects that has taken place, but also of necessary reciprocal support to guard against collapse.[24] Such support, however, presupposes the closure of the houses and the invisibility of the life they contain. Adele's specification of this speaks to a containment function that cannot completely relate to difficult emotions – a representation that emphasises more a defensive closure than the use of doors and windows as pathways of permeability.

In the closed and tightly overlapping houses, one can discern an attempt to dramatise, and thus to communicate through play, a feeling of "uncanniness"[25] present in the analytic field that one glimpses in the chaotic juxtaposition of Lego blocks. From another point of view, however, the playtime construction with Legos makes me think of the necessity and the analytic task of constructing or expanding the container through multiple experiences of connections, before unconscious contents can be confronted.

The fantasies, dreams, myths, and artistic creations, the images introduced into the field by the child as well, are a basic, symbolically protected area for the psychic transformation of raw, undigested emotions and the growth of the mental container. In this sense, I consider my associations to Schiele's work not only as my thoughts but as a further partial working-through of the thoughts present in the group.[26]

> It could fall to a specific individual to have the capacity to formulate the thought or the idea. But I don't think that the actual germination of the idea is attributable to a specific individual. It is very difficult to localize the phenomenon.
> (Bion 2005, p. 117)

In the attempt to catch hold of something in the lump of emotions that circulate in this little family group, I think of the houses painted by Schiele in the brief period between 1911 and 1913 in which he moves to Krumau, his mother's birthplace. In this part of Bohemia, the subjects of his paintings are primarily representations of houses without any people. As evidence of those who inhabit the houses, there are only clothes hung outside to dry[27] (see Figure 3.1).

These paintings of the Krumau houses allow me to see that sometimes loneliness can be juxtaposed without communicating. But in the detail of the clothes hung out to dry, I recover the hope of possibly revealing intimate emotional elements to the other, emotional elements that unite all human beings – just as laundry does. Furthermore, present in the hanging clothes is the faith that warmth from outside can dry them.

I share Adele's play with her dad, describing it in a Skype session in which both parents are present. In talking about the closed houses, we share the anguish of isolation that we are all experiencing and the loneliness it entails for Adele and for all of us. The dad underlines the non-tragic nature of a separation that will have an end, and by contrast he allows into our discussion the presence of a loneliness following the loss of a parent – the incredulity of abandonment and the rage that follows from it. This is an emotion known to his wife in relation to the loss of her friend, about whom she again speaks with great pain. Both parents try very hard to keep this suffering hidden, confined to memory, but it now resurfaces in connection with the forced separation.

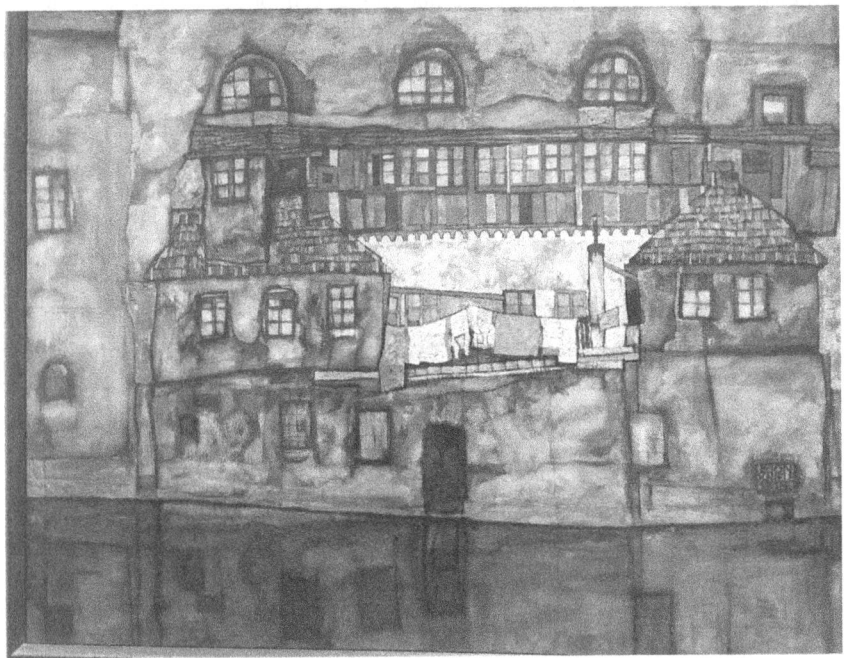

Figure 3.1 E. Schiele's *House Wall on the River*.

I emphasise that in her play, Adele alternates moments of construction with those of relative destruction and difficulty in putting the Legos back together. I say:

Analyst: She, too, is having experiences of how difficult it is to put the pieces back together after having destroyed the houses. Her hands are not yet expert, and it might be that precisely in facing a similar experience, she might try to obtain pleasure for herself.

Both parents are moved by their daughter's difficulty and seem to better understand the meaning of her resort to masturbation. Towards the end of the session, they decide not to give away the turtle for which Adele seems to have developed an affection. In this session, through Adele's play, the parents gain access to a greater awareness of the losses, scarcely worked through, that both have suffered, and in the decision not to get rid of the turtle, one sees an increased capacity to master the split, the withdrawal and the sense of persecution that accompany them.

Three women in one: the sister, the lover, and the wife

Adele and her mom keep in daily contact with the dad through Skype. Initially, the husband tells of all the pain he witnesses, and in particular the agonising farewells of some of his patients who say goodbye to their loved ones before dying during a video call. This detail calls to my mind an interesting observation made by Resnik in an article entitled "The Hands of Egon Schiele" (2000). Resnik examines a locomotive drawn by the painter at the age of ten years, and in the smoke it emits, he identifies the trace of a hand (see Figure 3.2).

Schiele was the son of a station master, and according to Resnik's reconstruction, he witnessed daily the separations between those who left and those who stayed, fixating on the painful gesture of the waving hand – and on something of his own difficulties with separation as well. Such difficulty was aggravated by the

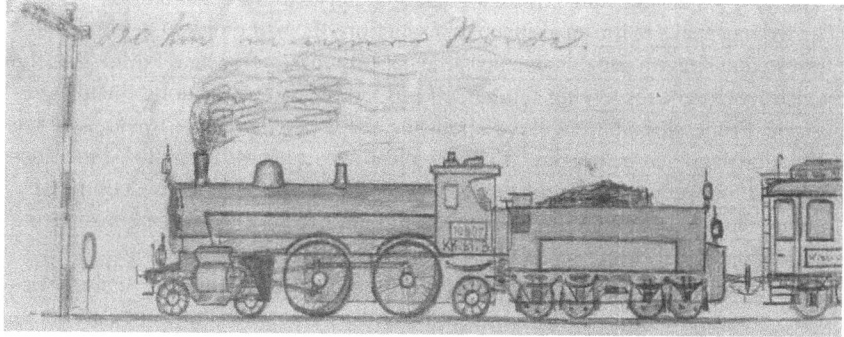

Figure 3.2 Locomotive with smoke. Schiele's drawing made during his childhood.

death of his father from syphilis when Egon was 15 years old, after some years of psychiatric disturbances due to the cerebral localisation of the illness.

A somewhat surprising aspect of the evening conversations between husband and wife is that, after an initial phase marked by painful stories, the husband begins to get seductive, displaying his erotic desire in a completely new and explicit manner. It is not unusual that persons immersed in seriously traumatic and lethal situations cling to life through Eros, but initially the woman was scandalised by this and judged her husband severely. She talks to me about it in a session in which Adele is not present. I tell her:

Analyst: It happens in a couple that each can be for the other a parent or a sibling, but discovering the lover in the other person is a healthy aspect, even if this emerges in an unusual way.

I say this thinking about how Schiele used his much-loved sister, Gertrude, as a model, portraying her in decisively erotic poses – to the point that he met with the 17-year-old Walburga Neuzil, known as Wally, who depicted a great many sexually explicit poses, including masturbation.[28]

Perhaps feeling some minor resistance on his wife's part, the husband's desire becomes ever more daring, until one evening he asks her to take off all her clothes and to become aroused by touching herself. Adele's mom is very annoyed by this and is consumed by fantasies that her husband may be attracted to another woman; certainly, she is not the lover whom her husband desires. Categorically, she will not do certain things, and she feels wounded by being treated like a prostitute. Deep inside, her rage and displeasure grow at a dizzying rate – to the point that, for some days, she feels compelled not to answer calls from her husband on her cell phone or on Skype.

Thus, a very painful situation of loss of contact is created in both of them. The separation they suffer, at the moment not resolvable in a meeting, reactivates in each of them the echo of a mourning not fully worked through. The husband sends a storm of messages to the wife in which he asks her forgiveness, pleading the innocence of his desires and expressing anger at her extreme reaction.

The woman seeks in me an alliance that sanctions the pathology of her husband's request so that she can use this in a possible petition for divorce, and I think that she may also feel angry for having felt herself pushed by my words along this dangerous slope. Somewhat apprehensive about the unexpected wrinkle towards which the situation seems to be heading, the only clear aspect seems to me to be the non-coincidence between the form of the father's erotic desire and Adele's compulsive symptom. But about this assumed connection I am not yet capable of constructing a communicable narration.

The hypothesis of holding a session with the couple together is scarcely doable for practical reasons; furthermore, I vividly remember the father's embarrassment when the wife had verbalised his nail biting during our earlier sessions. The emergence of the erotic theme, narrated in an overly explicit way, risks producing a fracture.

Feeling somewhat responsible for not having been attuned to a register of tolerating the emotions at play, I think that my breakdown in providing effective psychic help may be located at the intersection of many levels in this familial group: the therapeutic one, the historical one, and that in relation to Adele. Like me, the parents cannot have been capable of offering sufficient containment and emotional synchronisation with Adele, who finds herself alone in managing an excessive quantity of pain that she tries to remedy by getting pleasure from masturbation.

I am also apprehensive about the emergence of an erotic turbulence that momentarily shores up the difficulty of getting through pain. I say to the mom:

Analyst: I don't think that your husband had the intention of putting you in difficulty or dangerously exposing you. Sometimes exaggerating the wish to look hides the desire to be looked at.

After a silence, I add:

Analyst: You had your friend with whom your feelings were truly mirrored. Maybe your husband seeks something similar in you.

As I speak these words, a possible connection is clarified for me between the two subjects that predominate in Schiele's work: the self-portrait and the erotic representation of his models' bodies. They can be seen as two sides of the same desire: looking and being looked at passionately. Outside the session, I reflect on the fact that to undertake a self-portrait, artists often make use of a mirror, and Schiele, too, painted his by using – at least initially – the very mirror that had been given to him by his mother when he was sixteen years old, on the occasion of her departure for Vienna's Academy of Fine Arts in 1906. Having been orphaned the year prior to painting the self-portrait, Schiele clings to this mirror as though it could represent the maternal eyes in which he is reflected. This experience was mostly unknown to him as he was growing up because of his mother's difficulties in being with him during his early childhood and then again in adolescence, in that she herself was burdened by grief and difficulty related to her husband's illness. A "dead" mother, psychically, is thus agonisingly sought after in a compulsion for self-portraiture.[29] The relation to eyes that gaze lovingly plays out for Schiele in the relationship with his sister, and then with other, subsequent models, in an increasing capacity for distancing from the familiar. The counterpoint between the events in Adele's family and Egon Schiele's work is obviously an arbitrary element but a useful one for transforming emotional upsets into images.

The woman doesn't comment on my reference to the intimate confidentiality and mirroring with her friend, a relationship that seems to precede formation of the birth of the third, understood as psychic space in the meeting with the other-than-the-self, toward which the husband is pushing her through the erotic relationship[30]. She agrees, however, to an evening Skype call with her husband. Adele's mom gradually allows herself to be seduced in the dialogue with her husband – not to the point of concretely undressing but liberating herself from inhibitions about speaking of the desire to get out of the suffocating role of caregiving to which her husband, too, contributes to incarcerating her.

After a little while, the husband comes home, and he, too, manages to open up about the pain and anger that have been held inside him for many years, never finding a means of expression except through his body, in the desire to tear off tiny pieces of skin from his fingernails. One can imagine that, beyond the normal young sexual impulse, the tragic events of life spurred Adele's dad to seek pleasure and consolation in masturbation during his youth, more so than what normally happens.

Schiele writes in his diary:

> Have adults forgotten how it was for them as little ones? How they were pushed and also lifted up by the sexual impulse? Have they forgotten what terrible passion burned within them and tortured them when they were children? I myself have not, I have not forgotten, because I suffered terribly from it.
>
> (A. Roessler, ed., cited by Comini 2018, p. 42)

Only the forced separation resulting from the pandemic has brought back to the surface the old way of confronting first the mother's loss and the father's a little later, rendering the audacious request made to the wife a kind of waking dream in which there is a basis both of the pleasure of the body that comes from masturbation and of the mental pleasure that comes from looking and being looked at by the mother. The computer screen employed during the video calls perhaps played a role in creating this mirroring effect and a distance/closeness that was useful in inducing greater freedom of thought and word.

Paradoxically, in a scenario where death seems to dominate, this couple finds the words with which to relate to each other more intimately, to transform distance into closeness, to invent for themselves a new pattern of intimacy within the couple. In parallel to a new framework for desire and for the exploration of pleasure in more adult ways by the parents, the problem of Adele's masturbation was attenuated, to the point that it appeared only occasionally and in a way more in keeping with her age.

Seeing and being seen

To see, which is also a tool for knowing, is a function that is physiologically quite deficient at birth. Binocular vision is a complex function that is refined in the first two years of life and fully established only at around the age of eight years. This is a pivotal point in development because it permits one to focus on details, to be aware of a certain portion of space and of its depth, and to utilise vision in the service of action. At the same time, it is an event that intersects with the development of knowledge, of awareness and of ideas.[31]

If we transfer this premise into the analytic relationship, what does *seeing* mean – seeing and focusing, being aware of what happens in a certain portion of space, and knowing how to use this information? How can we intuit and thus see the unconscious interweaving of relational connections and symptoms, and especially how can we share this in the family group?[32] The starting assumption is that here, too, as in individual therapy, in family treatment there is not a subject who thinks and one to whom the meaning of what is said or done is communicated (interpreted). In the Bionian perspective, thinking is not done inside the subject but is always, from the beginning, a relational piece of data. Just as seeing stereoscopically requires two eyes, thinking requires two subjects.

In the relationship with a very small child, beta elements – which constitute the initial legacy of the child's bodily sensations – become perceptions that have a meaning merely by passing through the alpha function of the other, which actually thinks them with him. In this early phase, if we want to set up a parallelism with the visual function, it is possible to say that mother and child are trying to learn how to put sensation and emotion together in order to capture simultaneous images. In biological vision, each eye sees an image, and in order to avoid doubling, it is necessary to learn a way of coordinating that guarantees the perfect superimposition (fusion) of what each eye sees. Analogously, one can say that every time mother and child understand each other emotionally, which successfully focuses their respective feelings/emotions in the here and now, the two of them reach an emotional unison that creates an affective pictogram (an alpha element). Over time, the production of many alpha elements allows the structuring of a function (the *contact barrier*[33]), which generates an early distinction between the conscious and the unconscious. At the beginning, everything is conscious; it is sensation and perception. The unconscious is created in the relationship of two subjects who manage to focus on and share an emotion; the term *binocular vision* describes the rapport between these two parts of psychic functioning.

The possibility of having the experience of a group relationship, such as, for example, that of the family, can be an occasion to see in greater depth or more clearly something that is beyond normal perceptive capacity – a way to approach comprehension of parts of the self that are otherwise inaccessible.[34] These are protomental states, elements that get registered in a sensorial way and are not spontaneously directed toward signification – forms of procedural memory, implicit or not declared, early traumas that get deposited in the body, in a memory without recollection.

One could say that within a group therapeutic framework, the possibility of tridimensional vision is generated, a vision that is deeper and more clear. In biology, tridimensional vision is the result of a very complex integration imposed by the necessity of mastering the distance between the two eyes. This distance would generate perceptive distortions were there not an intervention from a system not so much acting as a corrective (as happens for the fusion of the images of the two eyes), but instead as a system that can learn to integrate different information that correlates memory with many associative areas of the cortex. Psychic learning, which permits tridimensional vision in a network of conscious and unconscious relationships, sometimes starts from a fracture in this network: the malaise of a group member. In a family, not infrequently, this malaise converges in a child's symptom, that of a particularly sensitive subject whose psychic immaturity creates the availability of being a container of a malaise that is not only the child's own.

The symptoms manifested by a child activate in the parents the desire and attempts to take care of the symptom, but also defensive emotional reactions, sometimes primitive ones, and wild thoughts.[35] Wild thoughts[36] can be compared to the preconceptions of a small child – emotions, affective states, basic wishes that must be thought. In the case of the group, however, wild thoughts – unstructured ones, unconnected to other thoughts – are often uncomfortable, aggressive, shameful. Although called thoughts, they are not fully such because they take on a form in which the physical and the psychic exist in an undifferentiated state.[37] Such thoughts generate a sort of contagion among the group's components and continue to circulate until the collective alpha function renders them thinkable and thus speakable. In this situation, too, it is the *trans-individual* who thinks, not the single mind. The possibility of focusing on a wider, tridimensional vision, which is generated in considering the relationship between the subject and the group, has been described by the term *binocular vision* – not by chance the same expression used to describe the conscious-unconscious relationship.

Just as the conscious and the unconscious become the products of a gradual differentiation carried out by the alpha function, the group's components become fully formed subjects to the degree to which each becomes aware of and masters his or her own emotions. In the group analytic field, a valid paradox exists: the greater the emotional identity of each component, the healthier is the relational connection. In other words, the more the parents take possession of their own emotions, the more the child has the possibility of developing without the burden of undigested emotions that are not the child's own.

The analyst's role: a corrective lens

Which method can the analyst use in a family or group field to help each of the subjects focus on their own emotions and distinguish them from those of the others? In the past fifty years, various methods of treating the child's difficulty in relation to that of the parents have been developed.[38] Those methods, like differing corrective lenses, propose different areas of focus in the therapeutic process. Some authors particularly concentrate on the child's internal world and that of the parents, while others place emphasis on supporting the parental function. Almost all attribute a crucial role to the child, agreeing that use of the child's nonverbal communication can improve the process.

Such a common position, however, is newly opened wide in the answer to the question of whether the child is considered a subject who participates in the process and in what way, or whether he or she is merely influenced by it. The answer implies a different theory of technique. One option is for the therapist to focus on the child's unconscious needs and to communicate directly with the child[39]; a different option is to consider the child's suffering as a result of the mother's or father's unconscious conflict. In this case, the analyst does his or her best to put the unconscious traumatic memories of one of the parents into contact with the child's symptoms.[40] A third possibility is to consider the family as a small group in which the child's symptom represents – in addition to a difficulty – the possibility for each subject to move toward a psychic transformation that allows him/her to approach a level of optimal subjectivisation. This technique involves focusing not only on suffering located in the past but also on its reproduction in the present, in the analytic situation. Considering the emotional interaction among subjects, it is possible that the analyst concentrates on grasping how an emotion may be shared among the group's subjects. Focusing on emotional unison reactivates, to a certain degree and at a group level, the initial pattern of the mother-child relationship, when reverie allows the child to recognise his or her own emotions in identification with the mother's feelings, and such identification permits the birth of the psyche out of the body. In other words, this emphasises an identification of feelings between two or more components of the group, as the place in which each subject's difference comes into being and is given shape.[41] Recognising the emotion present in the intersubjective field and correlating it to the events of the analysis is what Bion calls "being in unison with O" in the session. Since O cannot be grasped with the intellect, to be receptive to the intersubjective unconscious level involves not only an observation of the interaction but also listening to the unconscious. "Speculative imagination" is a faculty of the mind that can create a common field between the field of imagination and that of comprehension, two areas that Freud maintained are distinct but that Bion places in relation to each other through identification of their common space.[42]

The role of the child as a subject of the little group (parents-analyst-child) is that of one who is more capable than the others of activating the imagination, especially through play, and of drawing attention to some of the sensorial and aesthetic elements. The child is thus able to support the upward surge of usable images from the imagination and then eventually to transform them into a communication. The embodied experience of the child's symptom, then, can be considered the beginning of a potential space between perceptive experience and reflective experience, for each member of the group.[43]

The child as an erotic resource

Eros, in its Greek root, has not only the connotation of sexual attraction but is also understood as a force that contains different though united elements, and sometimes these elements conflict but without reaching the point of being dissolved.[44] In the Greek pantheon, the god Eros is the only divinity represented as a child – first a young man and then a small child who has been provided with a bow and arrow with which he can strike the heart of whomever he wants to make fall in love. Transferring this representation to the analytic situation, it is possible to think that, within the family, children represent the subject capable of introducing into the field arrows of "wild thoughts" that must in some way be transformed, thereby pushing those around them toward new thoughts. Wild thoughts, neither structured nor connected to other thoughts, are often uncomfortable, aggressive and shameful.[45] They are such because all ideas, before being thought, are a mixture of elements that no subject alone can handle. But because this may arise, it is necessary for the group together to reach the point of thinking what none of the members is capable of doing alone.

During the treatment of a child with his or her family, it is possible both to concentrate on the particular relationship between the child and the parents, and to emphasise attention to the group dynamics that flow through the family and into which the therapist enters to take part. One could say that oscillation between an analytic vision centered on the here and now of the relationships among the various subjects of the family, on the one hand, and the family as a group, on the other, is possible only in an erotic field – a field pervaded, that is, by passion and coupling without destroying the existence of individual subjectivities.

Initially, a symptom appears in the child, and it is from here that the analyst can start out, allowing the malaise to remain placed within the body, until the germ of an idea is mature enough to be born.[46] The first stage of transformation of the symptom often coincides with the upward surge of an image into the field that brings with it an early feeling of consistency in the chaos of emotions, sensations that become more frequent and more pronounced in group meetings. If one considers the emergence of the chosen fact[47] and the aesthetic experience as aspects of a turning point in the process, one can hypothesise that, in a therapy, the child can play an active role in causing the emergence of an "aesthetic selected " fact – one that is also understood in the etymological sense of being connected to the senses.[48]

When one can make use of an image – not necessarily a shared one – the symptom is no longer only a manifestation of discomfort but also becomes the staging of a fantasy that inhabits it and transcends it. Furthermore, being able to consider the sexual fact in a broader imaginative context allows the passage from erotic desire to passion, a dimension more symbolic of the connection that permits "a dream, freed from space and time to move between individualities and generations".[49] With this family, then, one can say that: "Thinking is [has been] bearable only by its sensual component",[50] and that the little girl's arrows played an important role in the transformation of her parents' pain.

Notes

1 Freud intuited that the existence of unworked-through traumatic experiences can influence subsequent generations. The transfer of psychic torment into another person, in general an offspring, avoids the painful working through that a grandparent or parent is not capable of suffering through. This theme has been developed by many authors, such as Faimberg (1988), Eiguer (1997) and Imbasciati (2004).

2 Kaës (2009b) writes: "The unconscious is not entirely contained within the borders of individual psychic space. The psychic space of the connection is another location of the unconscious."

3 Novick and Novick 2013; Whitefield and Midgley 2015; Salomonsson 2015; Goodman 2017; Barish 2018; Alvarez 2018.

4 Bion 1962b.

5 *Astronomical seeing* refers to the amount of apparent twinkling of astronomical objects, such as stars, due to turbulent mixing in the earth's atmosphere, causing variations of the optical refractive index. The visual conditions on a given night at a given location describe how much the earth's atmosphere disturbs the images of stars as seen through a telescope.

6 Bion 1997b, p. 645.

7 Bion 1974, pp. 72–73.

8 Bion 1957.

9 Winnicott 1974.

10 Bion calls this phenomenon of obstacles to comprehension of emotional truth *inversion of perspective*. López-Corvo (2002) observes that Bion himself relates inversion of perspective to binocular vision.

11 Grinberg 1985; Harris 2011; Salomonsson 2012; Hinshelwood 2016.

12 "Sex is a name, but none of us 'sees' sex, though it is a word we often use" (Bion 1991, p. 206).

13 Billow 2000, 2003; Migliozzi 2016.

14 Bion 1963.

15 "When the mother loves the infant, what does she do it with? . . . My impression is that her love will be expressed by reverie" (Bion 1962b, p. 35).

16 This title is inspired by some photographs of Egon Schiele from 1914.

17 Only in retrospect did I realize that an aesthetic element that could have influenced my reference to Egon Schiele's artistic work might have been this initial cinematographic effect. Bonito Oliva (1984) writes: "Schiele's positioning is the consequence of a visual emphasis that utilizes a sort of framing that seems to predict cinema, as artificial and unnatural – shooting from above, examination from below or from the side, the foreground, a three-quarters view."

18 Schiele was an Austrian expressionist painter (12 June 1890 [Tulln an der Donau]–31 October 1918 [Vienna]).

19 According to Klaus Albrecht Schröder (2000), Schiele had had access to see the photographic monographs of hysterics observed by Charcot.

20 L. Pistiner de Cortiñas (2009) maintains that, in the therapist's mind, art has the same function as a womb that progressively generates in the patient the capacity to contain and transform.

21 In his final painting, *The Family*, done shortly before his death, Schiele depicts a young pregnant wife (in her sixth month) and her own death that occurred three days later. The baby who was never born is thus only imagined by the painter; it is represented by an ambiguous pose between birth and the squatting position of an older child between the maternal legs. The painting's overall composition harkens back to being contained within the other, as though to express the wish of every human being, not only of the child, to be contained by the body and mind of another.

22 Kaës 1994.

23 Eiguer 2004.

24 As defined by Kaës (2009b), unconscious alliances permit a group's subjects to reinforce in each member some of the processes or functions or pathological structures from which he/she obtains something beneficial to his/her own psychic stability.

25 The word *uncanny* in Italian loses its connection with the house. From a semantic point of view, the German term, *umheimlich,* is the opposite of *heimlich* (from *heim,* house); *heimlich* means comfortable, trusted, intimate, belonging to the house. Thus, *unheimlich* means unusual, foreign, unfamiliar. Freud also uses the term *unheimlich* to mean "confined to the house, hidden". Uncanniness is born when, in either an object or a situation, characteristics of otherness and familiarity are combined into a sort of "affective dualism" (Tricomi 2001).

26 One could say that "in thinking, we do not produce thoughts, but we grasp them" (Frege 1988, p. 68).
27 Cresti and Nannini (2014) describe Schiele's representation of houses in Krumau as "like a sterile mother, like a womb bereft of twentieth-century history still to come, an eroded womb from indifferent waters – ever more indifferent and cold." In addition, in the painting *The Dead Mother*, the artist represents even more explicitly the theme of a lack of maternal containment; here Schiele depicts a small child wrapped in the black cloak of his dead mother, as understood by Green.
28 In 1915, the relationship with Wally having been ruptured, Schiele marries Edith Harms, with whom he shares his life and art until 1918, when both die of the Spanish flu a few days apart.
29 As a testament to Schiele's frenetic activity, Fischer (1996) brings up the fact that Rembrandt, himself passionate about the genre of self-portraiture, at the age of twenty-eight years had produced only half the number of self-portraits painted by Schiele.
30 Winnicott 1989b
31 The word *idea* has its roots in the Greek etymon *eide,* to know, which in turn is rooted in a past tense of the Greek verb *orao,* to see.
32 Psychoanalytic intuition concerns being "able to 'see' the meaning" (Bion 1970, p. 223).
33 Bion 1962b, p. 100.
34 Bion (1961) postulates the existence of a third state of mind that defines *inaccessible.* He refers to proto-mental states as vestiges of physical events experienced by the fetus and in perinatal life – thalamic fears or sub-thalamic fears that have never had access to working through. The proto-mental system is represented as something in which the physical and the mental are located in a differentiated state.
35 Bion 1997b; Bolognini 1994.
36 *Wild thoughts* is a term with which Bion describes those thoughts that seem not to belong to us, that conflict with the rest of our personality, and that in groups seem to be transmitted to us by the mind of an other, almost without filter and without special carriers. In reality, these thoughts await placement in a wider thinking apparatus that can contain them and contextualize them.
37 "I have postulated the existence of a proto-mental system in which physical and mental activity is undifferentiated" (Bion 1952, p. 236).
38 Salomonsson 2014.
39 Norman 2004; Salomonsson 2007.
40 Fraiberg's (1975) term for unconscious maternal conflict deposited into the child is a *fantasma of the nursery.*
41 Kaës (1998) notes that we find ourselves confronting a psychic reality without a subject that would acquire autonomy, inevitably coming into being between subjects (the psychic space of intersubjectivity) and through subjects (the psychic space of transobjectivity).
42 Freud employs the term *Fantazieren* to speak of imagining and of Bildung to indicate the work of constructing concepts.
43 The bodily is itself a psychic event, even though in a form unknown to us (Freud 1940).
44 Ubaldo 2000.
45 Bion (1980) writes that wild thoughts are in the air, but no one has the courage to think them because they fear that they will be asked, "Why are you playing with that dirty idea?" (p. 201).
46 "Can we allow ourselves to seize the germ of an idea and plant it where it can be developed until it is mature enough to be born? We must not immediately expel the wild thought or the germ of an idea if we do not believe that it could survive if it were made public. When we make it public, it is then that we can give it a good look and decide whether to call it a memory or an intuition or a prediction or a prophetic statement, or even a sick germ" (Bion 1980, pp. 200–201).

47 Bion (1962b) described how, within the chaos of emotions and sensations that suddenly enter the field fast and furiously, an emotion can become more clear – becoming, that is, a chosen fact that permits a new feeling of coherence.

48 In *Transformations* (1965), Bion emphasized that when he thought of having captured the meaning of a symptom, it was often "by virtue of an aesthetic rather than a scientific experience" (p. 52).

49 De Toffoli 2014, p. 248.

50 Bion 1975, p. 159.

Chapter 4

Adolescent feminine subjectivities and the analyst's one

A creative crossing via transitory objects

In this chapter I seek to explore Winnicott's[1] concepts of the "masculine" and the "feminine" within the early mother-infant relationship in order to explicate how the masculine/feminine dimensions reappear in adolescence. Adolescence is a crossroad between the redefinition of the self and the cultures of the family and society. We also use Bion's concept of container/contained to examine the group dynamic of family and society that imagines the individual adolescent. The individual interrelates with the shared group unconsciousness and forms contexts of expectations and norms.[2] I also introduce the concept of "transitory objects" (discussed later in this section) as a way to capture and track shifting expressions of the masculine/feminine themes of an adolescent girl in analysis.

Winnicott uses the concepts of "masculine" and "feminine" not to describe the beginnings of sexuality but to describe the somatic relationship between mother and baby. He terms the "feminine element" as the earliest relationship between mother and baby, before the relationship with the object develops. The feminine correlates with "being", not excluding variation but otherness, and basically guarantees continuity of the internal and external environments. The "masculine element", on the other hand, has to do with an active relationship with the other and serves to recognise and accept differences. These elements have no relationship to gender; rather, they set up the paradox of relationality in their difference and, if not impeded, become a root of creativity. Winnicott[3] described the relationship between masculine and feminine as two distinctive but intimately connected elements, just as twins during gestation, though separate and different, brush against each other and lean on each other.

In this theoretical frame, the role of primary aggression is involved in the dynamic of recognising the "me" and the "not-me". In order for the object to be utilised and transformed from a subjective object into a true relational object, it must be able to be possessed, to be destroyed by the baby's innate aggression, and then to be re-created by him or her. This re-appropriation through aggression, which the object survives, forms the basis of the capacity to be in a relationship. Winnicott describes aggression as a basic element of psychic function from the origins of life through the concepts of "masculine" and "feminine". Aggression can play a positive, organising role during development, or, if characterised as a pathological element, can produce relational difficulties.

DOI: 10.4324/9781003388838-5

While Winnicott utilises the concept of masculine/feminine to describe the first steps of the mind in its impact with the world, Bion looks at the same relational dynamic and utilises the conceptual tool of the container/contained (♀ ♂) relationship. Bion describes the mouth/breast relationship and the psychic meeting between the mother's mind and the baby's mind through projective identification.[4] He focuses on the need for help from another mind to work through the negative feelings that emerge from frustration. The capacity to learn from experience is highly dependent on the availability of the container/maternal mind to accept projections. If this happens, the baby gradually internalises the capacity to contain his or her own mental states.

Bion also utilised the concept (♀ ♂) at a greater level of abstraction, applying it to the relationship between the subject and the group, whether familial or social.[5] At whatever level it is considered, the relationship of container/contained describes a dialectic essential to subjectivisation. Bion's interest is not so much in gendered sexuality as in the mental relationship between container/contained. However, he termed the relationship between container/contained "intercourse", thus maintaining its bodily roots.

The influence of gender intensifies in early adolescence as both internal and external demands require adjustment to changing circumstances. Adolescence is a liminal period when adolescents, their families and their psychoanalysts imagine the unfolding feminine/masculine theme. It is impossible to think of masculine and feminine separate from culture. We cannot, however, lose the concept of a subject who will organise experiences of biology and culture in a unique and not pre-determined form. In psychoanalysis, preconceptions about ourselves, including those related to gender, are examined and potentially reimagined by both patient and analyst. The tension between the culture-bound and the potential for new imaginings of gender may be an explicit or implicit theme of the work.

Adolescent sexual relationships co-construct and constitute versions of the feminine and the masculine. Such narratives of gender are compromise formations, which include over-determined normativities and yet are idiographic and embodied. Adolescents can ape cultural forms and yet simultaneously "try on" their own experiences. Conformity to cultural expectations leads to comprehensibility but threatens the unique and the personal. Boundaries of the "approved " have moved so significantly in contemporary culture that we constantly re-imagine gender.

I relate clinical material from a 14-year-old girl who came into treatment because her mother considered her behaviour towards her twin brother too aggressive. The family culture brought expectations about the behaviour of a young girl to the therapy. The presenting issue of the relationship between sister and brother introduced the male-female theme into the analysis, which was then present in the analytic relationship like a dream function. I use this clinical material to examine the way culture, family and psyche interweave in experiences of gender. I present an ongoing series of clinical moments between an adolescent girl and her female analyst and suggest that culture-bound experiences of the feminine are subtly reimagined in these moments.

Through the clinical material I also introduce the concept of "transitory objects". I use this term to describe drawings produced in the treatment built together by the analyst and the patient similar to Winnicott's squiggle technique. Transitory objects are relational tools able to promote the transition of self disconnection to connectedness. They have two sides: one that shows internal integration and a second one that shows the relational change. As Winnicott's squiggle, transitory objects condense in themselves the working-through of a process. In the current clinical work, they were used as a way to capture and track shifting expressions of the masculine/feminine themes of an early adolescent girl.

Child/adolescent analysis informs adult analysis through its emphasis on shapes and forms, which yield the beginnings of representability. This adolescent girl used artistic modalities to create visual representations that convey her emerging grasp of a complex unconscious masculine/feminine situation.[6] Play with a child or artwork with an adolescent can gather unprocessed beta elements into dream/alpha elements allowing the digestion of complex emotions. I describe a series of images that gave meaning to previously unthinkable emotions related to the feminine/masculine theme.

Winnicott contends that playing (or here artwork with an early adolescent) places both the psychoanalyst and the child in the moment at which things begin to take shape. This is synchronous with Bion's advice that the analyst: "abandons memory and desire (in order to be optimally intuitive and receptive to his own unconscious vis-à-vis the analysand)". Reflection and interpretation can occur after a period of the development of play/art experiences. The conception of transitory objects is also informed by the Barangers' (2008/1961)[7,8] assertion that the analyst's neutrality is impossible and that the patient and analyst are bound in a dynamic and complementary bi-personal field, a spatial and temporal structure with its own laws and dynamics, resulting from the joint creation of an underlying shared unconscious fantasy. What underlies this structure is a shared unconscious fantasy that is the product of unconscious communication and of a joint creation process. The clinical material presented will be followed by a discussion and then by a theoretical commentary that will include reflections on how our very attempts to redefine our concepts in relation to the masculine and feminine can still be trapped in old assumptions. I introduce "Violet" in her analyst's words.

Clinical case: Violet

Violet entered therapy at age 14 years because her mother felt that she was inexplicably overly aggressive toward her twin brother, in contrast to an equally excessive timidity and withdrawal in relation to others. The father, a silent and shy man, said that Violet looked like him and did not share his wife's concerns.

Violet's twin brother had not seemed to live up to their mother's expectations and was not very responsive to their mother's solicitations. As a younger child Violet had been at an advantage in satisfying her mother's needs. She maintained maternal approval until early adolescence as a good student and well behaved.

However, when Violet showed more open anger toward her brother at the beginning of adolescence (even though it was not much beyond a normal level of conflict between adolescent siblings), mother perceived her as intolerably aggressive. The mother was likely projecting a split part of her own unconscious hatred towards her disappointing male child. The mother's difficulty in taking care of two children (not only in a concrete manner) may be shown by the fact that a nanny still lived with the family even now that the twins were mid-adolescents.

I describe the first two years of her twice weekly treatment.

My meetings with Violet always took place in the room used for therapy with children and adolescents, a larger one than the room where I work with adults, and with a table for playing or drawing. Since the entryway accesses both therapy rooms (which are on opposite sides), if the doors are not properly closed whoever enters can easily glance into one or the other room. Soon after our meetings began, Violet asked me if she could look at the room that she glimpsed on entering – where, she said, "(W)e never go in."

I acquiesced, and we sat on the chairs there for some minutes, close to each other. She observed a series of little paintings on slabs of solidified limestone, which I had done during my analysis. The paintings represented women who, in all probability, embodied parts of me that were in transformation. For some years, I had kept them concealed, like products of a relationship that was too intimate to be shown, but eventually, it seemed to me that they were entitled to a place that represented an ideal continuity between the room where I had done analysis as a patient and the new one where I practiced as an analyst.

Violet's attention was attracted by two of my paintings:

Violet: This woman seems lonely.

Then, she fixed her gaze on another painting (see Figure 4.1).

Violet: This one, in contrast, seems to be a ballerina, like me. . . . in a trap.

Her remarks had the effect of arousing in me a cluster of memories, reflections and emotions that seemed not to have been tamed much either in my analysis or in the paintings. Although it may seem absurd, I had never really thought about how my not having been able to pursue dancing (for various reasons that were difficult to accept) had become merged with the tunic with which I had dressed the "imprisoned" woman. The "imprisoned " ballerina was thus an image of my very early feeling of not being able to move or to rebel.

The other painting, the only one on a different mounting, represents an adult woman, nude, curled up tightly as though contained in a uterine sphere. Geometric, angular forms take up half the oval stone on which it is painted, in stark contrast to the other elements that resemble a biological setting. To be in contact with the angular parts of one's own mother or of one's analyst, and to be trapped, now appeared to me as elements of relating to each other with a new rapport. When

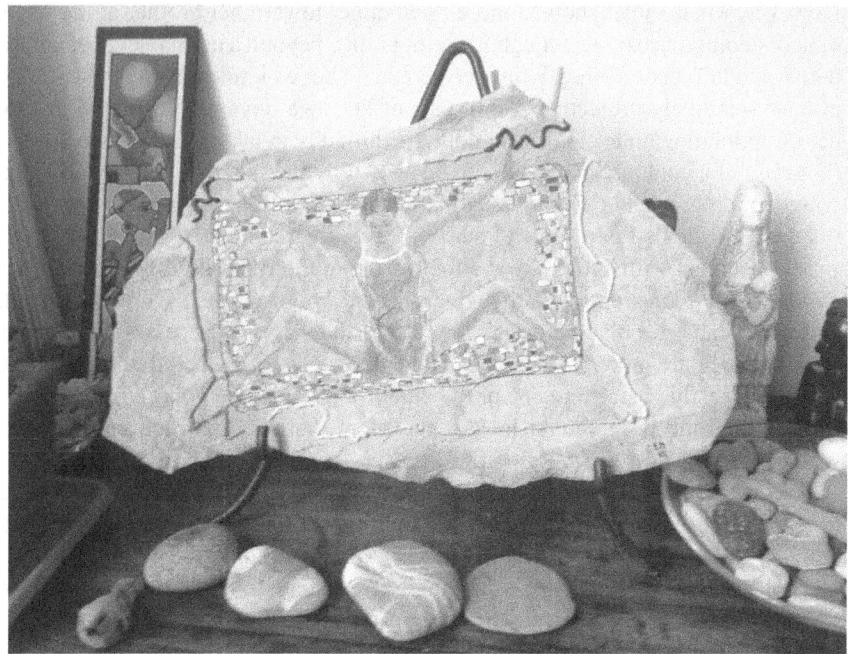

Figure 4.1 E. Molinari, *Solitude in the Mirror*.

we returned to our usual room, Violet wanted to begin to paint, using some plastic materials.

The artistic objects that marked the stages of our journey – I consider "transitory objects" (discussed further later) – are objects created by Violet and by me.

I present the work with this young girl in three segments.

Doors: transition and borders of setting

My association to Violet's wish to go into a forbidden room – or to open a closed door – was to the doors implemented by Kunellis in Sarajevo right after the end of the conflict in the former Yugoslavia. These doors were filled in with various concrete materials that completely obstructed transit: books, bells, sacks etc. These materials transformed doors from architectural elements indicating passage to elements that enclose and entrap, becoming symbolic of what conflict can produce: a reduction of tri-dimensionality to life in a flat and potentially lethal space.

My decision to allow Violet to enter the adult room was a response to her desire to enter a "new place," as in a different relation with me. The memory of Kunellis's exposition pushed me not to obstruct the possibility of a development with theory and a rigid application of the setting. I was aware that the frustration of Violet's desire would allow a limit and anger about frustration with the possibility of transforming emotions with words as usual in the therapeutic setting. However, current developments in the psychotherapeutic treatment of adolescents suggest that the setting may be used in a more flexible way as a therapeutic factor given the adolescent desire to change the setting in relation to their development. Although adolescents need containment that gives them a sense of solidity and continuity, they also need a tailor-made setting, not the application of anonymous rules. Transforming the setting in a shared space allows the teenager to feel not only involved but co-responsible. Adolescents don't like to feel as passive subjects of an investigation showing their weaknesses and pathology but as subjects whose therapy offers the opportunity to transform difficulties into a demanding self-exploration.[9]

Violet asked me for stones similar to the ones I had painted on to continue to share and explore this new place we had entered. Not having any at our disposal, we decided to spread some little wooden tables with soft dough made of sand and glue, in order to create a surface similar to the backing of my paintings.

Over the course of several sessions, these little tables came to be carved into and scratched with various tools without the end result of any particular representation. In engaging in this project, Violet displayed a mixture of courage and inhibition: she felt able to transmit her rage through this activity. At the same time it frightened her to a degree that she continually asked for confirmation that what she was doing was right. My approval was indispensable to her to discover her capacity to express her feelings in this external form, but my refraining from giving advice, as usual in the analytical setting, also allowed Violet to be pleasurably surprised by her results. This work together with non-symbolic signs was similar to the squiggle play of Winnicott, a way to be in relationship able to introduce the experience of reciprocity: "me a little and you a little".[10,11]

So, we decided to color the tables, and once they were dry, to put water on them to remove any excess and create a more variegated effect. The result was one of surprising beauty: the aggressive action now represented something rising up, far from the stereotype of destruction. The dough made of sand and glue that had lent support now seemed to have a soul capable of accepting and modulating the intensity of the color, mimicking in the material the functions of the maternal psychic container. The possibility of actively correcting the result through jets of water legitimised the expression of something that seemed excessive; modulating the saturation of color thus became a gesture that could restore to her, at least partially, the legitimacy of her feelings.

We talked about the work as it gradually began to take shape, and also about Violet's fear every time something inconvenient happened. Going beyond the edges of the dough or the drips of glue on the table sometimes caused Violet to freeze, manifested at times as indifference and at other times an excessive worry. When I felt able to introduce the topic of reactions to what occurred more explicitly – particularly the anger – Violet spoke for the first time of her difficult relationship with her brother (mother), who she felt did not know how to respect limits and continually invaded her space.

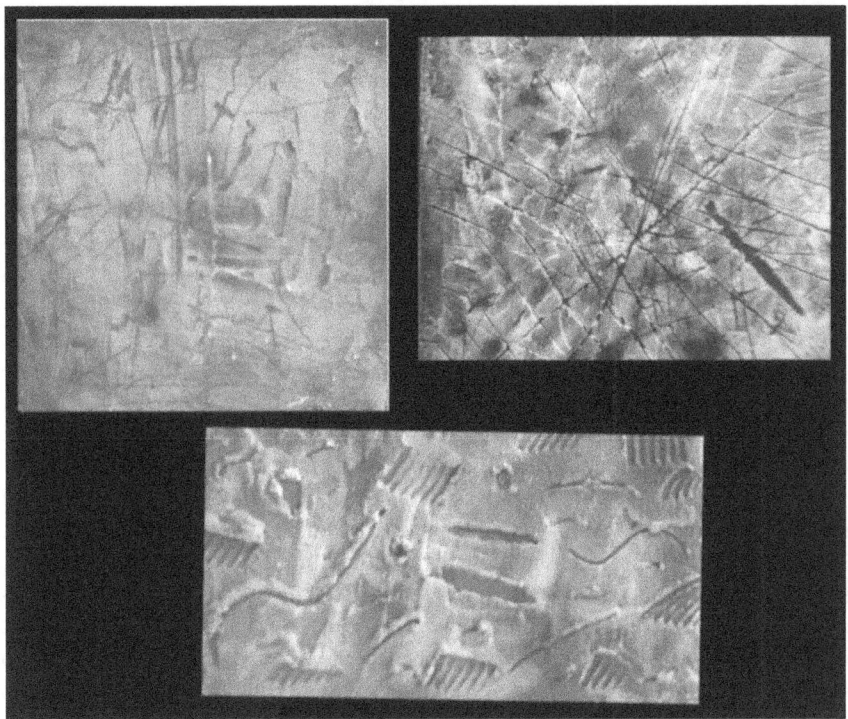

Figure 4.2 Violet's scratching drawings.

I thought that Violet's conflict with her brother helped her to legitimise her rage toward her mother, felt in the past as rather inaccessible. In the present her rage helped her understand her feeling shut out of her maternal relationship in failing to conform to their mother's expectations.

I thought that having allowed Violet to enter the adult therapy room and experience reproducing and transforming something of mine, scratching and coloring it and then erasing part of the color, must have also had an impact on the psychic process in being. I thought that Violet might have experienced a new relationship with her internal mother, able to experience both the "feminine" aspects of being one and the "masculine" aspects of being active and different from the other (see Figure 4.2).

Selfies: at a cross-road with the analyst's culture

After about a year, as she spoke of selfies that she and her friends loved to exchange via social media, Violet suddenly and without connection to our conversation asked me a very disconcerting question:

Violet: The pictures in the other room – are they your selfies?

Jokingly, I answered that they could be Paleozoic selfies adapted to someone of my age, given that they were painted on stone. But inside I asked myself how she could have raised this question without knowing that I had painted the images. She laughed at my response, but evidently she had noticed my surprise and the emotions that had flashed through me. To reinforce and not renounce her intuitive perception, she added:

Violet: The woman inside the frame, looks like you.

The figure represented did not look like me at all, and I had never thought of doing a true self-portrait, but the starting point from which I had taken the idea for the frame/prison had been a mirror. I said nothing of this, of course, but it upset me that Violet was so closely in contact with something of mine and remembered so precisely what she had seen for only a few minutes a year earlier.

Violet proposed a return to painting in order to show me something she had learned at school during art class. She took a sheet of paper and used Scotch tape to delineate a series of stripes. Then she painted some irregular squares with a sponge, wanting to use pink and purple for her colors, and at the end she took away the tape.

Violet: Look, it looks a little like your frame.
Analyst: So this is sort of a selfie of yours.

This picture inaugurated a period of investigation and reflection about borders of the self and those between self and other, and how "to be annoyed" makes relationships difficult – or sometimes it can tear them apart, as had happened with the support of the paper when the tape was torn off.

Violet: A less adhesive Scotch is needed – paper Scotch, for example.

This expression is a nice layman's definition of what Bion calls the "invariant": the possibility that between transformations brought about by the analyst (T_a) and those brought about by the patient (T_p), one can find an emotional continuity that guarantees the understanding and development of the psychic container.[12]

The use of two colors near each other from a chromatic point of view (pink and purple) and their clear distinction through white lines can be seen as an aesthetic investigation into the experience of continuity and separation. In addition, the tears in the supporting paper highlighted how Violet's rage produced analogous painful tears in the affective continuity with her mother, and how these exposed her to gradually feeling herself fragile and incapable.

Wanting to preserve her work, Violet then passed a layer of transparent glue over the surface, which gave it brightness and textural consistency, reaffirming that greater closeness guarantees solidity. We spoke in the concrete, of course, but reflection on how the same kinds of materials (paper on paper) could better relate to each other – just as how anger (getting annoyed) could produce holes – went beyond technical aspects. To be united, to be separated, to stick together, and to be torn apart, through action, assumed a dimension of great depth. Violet found it impossible to criticise her mother during this phase of adolescence, choosing her brother as the target of her aggressiveness. Her sense of solitude and lack of value did not permit her to move about fluidly in her feminine and masculine parts. Moreover, the stigmatisation of her aggressiveness as intolerable deprived her of the experience of containment in the family context. Violet felt left alone by a mother who projected into her daughter her own unthinking anxieties. Her father had difficulty in taking an active role, and her brother had become the object of her aggression.

Nail polish: the feminine at a cross-road with the family's culture

A third phase of the working through of these themes occurred through Violet's passion for nail polish and for makeup in general. Makeup was a battlefield with her mother, who countermanded her requests not only with prohibition but also with a moral judgment about her femininity. Violet wanted to strengthen her nails and at the same time beautify them, almost to the point of setting up inside herself the paradox of wanting and not wanting to use her aggression to differentiate herself from her mother. Moreover, the painted nails gave her a feeling of belonging with her group of friends.

One day, Violet arrived for her session with some bottles of nail polish that she had acquired in earlier months, but – not being able to use them or not feeling that she could legitimately use them – she found that merely looking at them aroused intense anger in her. She asked me if I would keep them until she decided to pour them down the toilet. Why empty them into such a specific container and not simply throw them away? In analysis, Violet sought a container for a part of herself that was considered unacceptable. At the same time she did not want to be impulsive and collude with the maternal judgment that nail polish (and anger) had to be likened to excrement. She wanted our relationship to be capable of representing a temporary lapse of time that was useful for understanding.

Violet tried to paint her nails in my consulting room, as though she might have a place in which to transgress. Her difficulty of using her left hand (the smudging due to the non-dominant hand's motoric imprecision) brought her to intense anger in the session. I felt this impossibility of her hands being interchangeable as a bodily representation of the feminine and the masculine, that only with difficulty find a psychic balance when adverse relational or cultural events impede their original capacity to coexist.

In subsequent sessions, Violet wanted to do experiments with nail polish. She let liquid from the little bottles drip onto a sheet of paper like drops of blood, creating a mark that she then shaped with a stick, as though to test its consistency.

We next filled a sink with water, and Violet emptied the bottles of nail polish, creating a marbled liquid image. She told me that it looked like a screen saver on her cell phone that she liked, an image she wanted to "capture" with the help of a sheet of paper.

Her association with a screen saver implied to me a cross-road between her need to use her phone to be in contact with her friends and her existence within her family.

The marks that emerged on paper were satisfactory and surprising, and the aesthetic effect of their combination appeared to her to be an instance of "getting on well together". She chose to hang some pink ones and some dark blue ones from a series of these works, lining them up together in a regular way. The colors made me think again of gender and of the pink and blue bows that are hung on the outside of a front door when there has been a birth. Violet's works appeared to me to represent the birth of a possible balance of the masculine and the feminine within her and a newly born desire to be able to show this accomplishment to the outside world.

"Transitory objects"

The unique feature of the therapeutic journey with Violet was that we were able to meet in an intersubjective field where something common to our subjectivation as females could be recognised and become useful in therapy. The beginning of a meaningful emotional transformation started through images present in my consulting room and then through other ones produced in the treatment.

Images root in the sensations more than words can. Images are the ground floor of identity and representation; for this reason I chose to describe the previous images as pivotal in redefining Violet's feminine identity as the treatment progressed. The use of painting was not primarily a way to explore feeling, as in art therapy. Rather, from a Field Theory perspective, the use of the images let Violet and me enter into a particular field of sharing.

The pictures described in the first phase of therapy allowed a state of sharing in which there was no distance, no clarity between here and there. Through Violet's first images about the body (evoked by my paintings), we started to explore something of primary femininity. These paintings produced by the patient and with the elaborations described earlier in the second and third phases of therapy, allowed us to explore the adolescent process. This redefinition expanded Violet's experience of gender identity including influences derived from her familial and societal gender culture.

In contrast to the "transitional objects" described by Winnicott (which represent a meeting between self and not-self and which define an area of play and illusion), "transitory objects" have the function of sketching out a sort of map between disorganising areas of self and their relational side[13]. They are "waking dream thoughts"[14] in the sense of a continuous transformation of raw sensations and[15] proto-emotions into narrative derivates. Objects with high sensory potential (such as plastic and color) are able to re-create a bodily and emotional transit, rich in sign and movement. Here, the creation of transitory objects permitted the integration of masculine and feminine parts of the patient and transformation of the therapeutic relationship as an external side of this integration.

The depths through the surface

The pathological connotation that Violet's mother attributed to her daughter's push to become a subject left Violet feeling marginalised in their relationship. This added a sense of growing frustration, of rejection of her own knowledge, to her original aggression. The social and cultural container, in addition to the maternal one, brought home to Violet that being aggressive was not appropriate to being female. This experience pushed her toward submissive behavior in social relationships. In addition to personal aspects, subsequent events (cultural or performative, as Butler defines them)[16] had widened the gap between the masculine modality and the feminine one of being in relation to the other.

The hypothesis of this contribution is that, when a cultural attitude that tends to pathologise the expression of feminine aggression is emphasised within the family, a specific alteration in psychic development results. Using Bion's symbolism, one can hypothesise that the missed experience of being contained in the mind of the other might produce a deformation in the development of the psychic container. In particular, stigmatisation of normal aggression as a pathological element produces in the adolescent an alteration in this psychic function, which manifests as confusion, an inability to decide, or a violent expulsion of rage through acting out. Through the previous material, I intended to show this psychic difficulty.

I also intended to show how some aesthetic tools, which I term "transitory objects", can be used, particularly in adolescence, to restore psychic functioning. Feeling marginalised has a double edge: the margins are where feelings of uncertainty or insecurity tend to flourish but may allow a creative point of view. Mother's projection into her daughter caused Violet to feel wrong for her mother – angry, uncontained and on the margins. The key question isn't how to eliminate this feeling but how to ride it. Transitory objects aren't necessarily art objects but relational tools able to promote the transition from the sorrow of relational disconnection to connectedness. This requires a deeper integration between feminine and masculine parts of the self.

From a Field Theory perspective, the analyst has to put aside the real relational story of the patient to focus on what happens between analyst and patient[17] (Ferro and Civitarese 2015; Molinari 2017). The flow of the transitory objects improved the capacity to transform sensations and raw emotions into waking dreaming.

Violet's artworks were not any artistic expression but were triggered by her analyst's paintings created during her own analysis, a very personal expression, captured by Violet with great sensibility. The way the patient can use the "objects" posed by the analyst and the opening of the analyst to offer part of her experiences, in a symbolic form, are moments of extreme fertility that reinforce our confidence in a non-omnipotent, sensitive psychoanalysis.

The old question of how the gender of the analyst helps or hinders the process is always present. This is not a simple question to answer, because it is not obvious that analyst and patient being of the same sex would facilitate the process. The fertility of the couple depends on many factors other than gender: the space offered and co-created, where feelings can be contained and find limits that allow them to be transformed in a non-accusatory climate. But, can we deny that femininity has its particularities that only two women can share? And that two men also share particularities?

Abandoning an old psychoanalytic view that might consider separation a goal of subject development, and observing the process that transitory objects allow, we can learn something more. We can observe how unconscious connections between minds – between individuals – determine what we know, how we know, and the vastly complex fields within which we affect each other in analysis and in culture. The images found in the analyst's studio and those produced by Violet represented, to a certain extent, a "subjective object" for each and at the same time the "thinking surface" of their meetings.

Violet's hatred toward her twin brother must not be understood as a simple relational difficulty but as rage at not feeling herself to be enough in the maternal mind. The maternal fear of that rage marginalised Violet compared to her brother, generating further demanding and violent behaviors, difficult to decode or to accept.

It can be posited that from the beginning, twins have different intrauterine experiences. Their preferred positions and interactions may also affect their relationship after birth. After birth, mother could give attention unconsciously more to one twin than the other. This can be due to a weaker baby or one that is more active. Each twin may be very jealous of the attention the other receives from their mother. Sometimes the access to maternal care being more difficult for twins strengthens the relationship between them so that over time they tend to consolidate complementary modes that produce a strong relationship. In other situations, particularly if mother struggles to maintain a balanced triangular relationship, the twins take on roles designed to meet maternal expectations and remain in competition with each other in a harsh way.[18,19,20]

Violet seemed to have taken on the mother's narcissistic sufferings and the angry disappointment toward the male twin. This did not allow her to internalise the male part, active and distant, integrating it with her own delicate, sensitive parts. She described her brother as intrusive and unable to respect limits.

Violet's difficulty seemed to root in an early stage of development of gender identity and relationship with the other. However, she was also on the threshold of adolescence, a time of life when the reshaping of the relationship with the parents and peers, as well as the influence of culture, had an important influence on the building of gender identity.

The therapeutic restitution of an experience of recognition, then, had to traverse two realms: the emotional one of anger and that of a relational practice aimed at modifying the "performative" or cultural aspects that influence gender identity, of which the parents are the natural means of transmission. Confusion and submission, in the final analysis, are the desire of the oppressed, and in this mother-daughter relationship, they are the epiphenomenon of the frustration of an intimate closeness. The non-acceptance of anger at a certain stage is shown to amputate the development of the container function, increasing projection as a defence.

Inclusion in the analytic relationship of an artistic experience and the creation of "transitory objects" permitted the integration of body and mind in the specifics of the therapeutic relationship with an adolescent. The aesthetic aspects belonging to the birth of the body-mind then functioned as vectors for the birth of little "affective padlocks," an expression of the social body-mind.[21]

Freud warned: "(I)t is important to understand that the concepts of feminine and masculine, whose meanings seem so free from ambiguities for ordinary people, are among the most confused in science."[22] Now, we know as the developmental processes intersect and interact with the subject's experiences of sexuality and desire, parents' wishes and culture; all these issues determine complex and changing gender identifications.[23] The clinical work presented here approaches the feminine/masculine subject starting from Winnicott's concepts of the creative constitution of the psyche. Winnicott contemplates the necessity of "being" (feminine) and "doing" (masculine) as essential elements for mental development. At the beginning of Winnicott's work, feminine and masculine are not directly related to gender; he used them in the same way Bion used feminine and masculine to refer to the container and contained[24]. Later, in his work *On the Split-off Male and Female Elements*,[25] he addressed the complexity of bi-genderness in psychic life and opened a new way of thinking about the process by which gender may emerge. In establishing first being and doing, sexuality becomes entangled with the parent's desire imbued with their conscious and unconscious subjective expectations. The possibility for traumatic effects is in the explicit messages sent to the child from the parents' projections and projective identifications.[6] We refer here to the thousands of teenagers who copy the protagonists of Federico Moccia's bestseller *I Want You* by attaching padlocks to bridges as a sign of eternal love. Enigmatic messages condition sexuality and identity during the developmental process. When these messages are massive and interfere with other features such as biological predisposition, the quality of attachment, or the presence of significant figures beyond parents, gender trauma[26] can result. The clinical case presented in this chapter doesn't show massive gender trauma. Rather, it allows us to see how the earliest mother and child links are an essential conduit for intergenerational transmissions about gender identity, as well as the impact during adolescence when the role of society become more relevant. Adolescence becomes a crucial time in development when the unconscious aspects of the parental message have a chance of transformation. But, of course, elements of these ongoing message transmissions were beyond Violet's mentalising capacities. Still, cognitive development, active sexual desire and the crucial task of differentiation make adolescence a time of possible retranslation of these messages. Psychoanalysis explores issues of gender and sexuality and how they shape the evolution of intersubjectivity. The immediacy of the immersive perceptive moment can allow embodied feeling states to emerge, where the gap between these forms and their context becomes crucial for new meaning. Contemporary psychoanalysis is as receptive to absence as presence and explores how presence is always an interplay between what becomes and what is not yet present. I tried to focus on the transformative point in which the intersection of the patient's and the analyst's experiences found boundaries and started going towards differentiation. Both the analyst and the patient had to do unconscious work to transform the understandable need for recognition which had been damaged by maternal projections. Transitory objects have been a helpful tool in the cross-road of personal and interpersonal re-creation of gender subjectivity.

Notes

1 Winnicott 1989a.
2 Bion 1961.
3 Winnicott 1989a; Ogden 2001.
4 Bion 1962b, 1970.
5 Brady 2018; Obholzer 1996; Grotstein 2013; Bion 1963.
6 Representability is also the work of adults in analysis, for instance, in integrating new experiences of pregnancy, aging or illness Such new experiences require emotional work to make meaning of them.
7 Bion 1967b, p. 136.
8 There are similarities between the Barangers and Italian Field Theorists such as Ferro, Civitarese and Molinari. For instance, Italian Field Theorists, e.g. Ferro 2002, particularly emphasize Bion's development of the importance of unsaturated interpretations and the continued creation of new meanings.
9 Laor 2007; Anagnostaki 2017; Ferro 2018.
10 Winnicott 2017b; Stefana and Gamba 2018 .
11 Winnicott, D. W. (1968). Playing: Its theoretical status in the clinical situation. *The International Journal of Psychoanalysis, 49*(4), 591–599.
12 Bion 1965, pp. 9–144.
13 Winnicott 1971a
14 Bion 1962b.
15 Butler defines *performative* as a repetitive act, anchored in culture, that renders gender norms unavoidable and ongoing. In this sense, culture would function with the same structural mandate as language (Butler 1990).
16 Kaës 2009a, 2010b
17 Piontelli 1989, p. 417.
18 Bion 1967a; Piontelli 2002.
19 Stewart 2003.
20 We refer here to the thousands of teenagers who copy the protagonists of Federico Moccia's bestseller *I Want You* by attaching padlocks to bridges as a sign of eternal love.
21 Freud 1905, p. 226.
22 Caldwell 2007; Chodorow 1989; Butler 1990; Benjamin 1998; Dimen 2003; Dimen and Goldner 2002; Corbett 2011, 2014; Harris 1997, 2002.
23 Bion 1971.
24 Bion 1963.
25 Winnicott 1989.
26 Saketopoulou 2014.

Chapter 5

Recognition takes a long journey

The protagonist of the *Odyssey* is a restless man who is married to a self-reflective woman.

Odysseus is the prototype of the man driven by an unquenchable urge to explore the world outside of himself, while his wife Penelope is left to cope with her own loneliness. Odysseus has many romantic adventures; Penelope lets other men court her, perhaps alternating between feeling flattered and rejected. Odysseus assumes a fatherly role towards his men; Penelope raises a fatherless child. The description of these two characters reveals the complementarity in how they function as a couple and, at the same time, as parents, as so often happens within the couple relationship. Becoming a father or a mother also means accommodating within the couple ghosts from their own childhood. This demands that both members of the couple embark on a long inner journey that enables them to put these spectres aside, become themselves and a real couple.

If we read the events narrated in the *Odyssey* as the story of a series of dreams, then we have the option of choosing whether or not to adhere to the narrative level that assigns the role of protagonist to one or the other of the characters.[1] I have chosen to focus on the chapters that describe Odysseus's encounters with a female character such as Calypso, Circe, the Sirens and Nausica, herein considered as partial aspects of femininity and different instances of becoming a couple.

The reunion between Odysseus and Penelope described in the final part of the poem may be considered not only as the epilogue of a journey that separated a man from a woman for 20 years but also as the discovery of a different kind of physical and emotional closeness within a couple who have faced the inevitable ups and downs of a relationship.

Each story of Odysseus's encounters with women is marked by twists and turns, adversity and pathos. This hidden tale became more evident to me whilst listening to the stories couples tell in therapy sessions. This is a reversal of the traditional approach which has been to use myths to illuminate life. Italo Calvino[2] writes:

> Odysseus is a modernly ambiguous figure, iridescent, "multiform", ingenious, as mobile as reality. In this case, it was the changing and multiform reality that made the tale of Odysseus and Penelope a prototype of life as a couple.
>
> (La Repubblica, 21.10.1981)

DOI: 10.4324/9781003388838-6

I therefore make use of some of the vivid stories I have heard in the consulting room to show how several of the episodes in the *Odyssey* can be rethought from the perspective of the ups and downs of life as a couple.[3] My aim here is not only to present a clinical case but to engage in a sort of literary rewriting of several universal issues.

"Enough, I am leaving": a modern version of the *Odyssey*

Giovanni and Beatrice arrive in the therapy room in the hope of averting a separation, both driven by a sense of responsibility towards their two children. What is making the attendant pain and relational tension all the more intolerable is the measure Giovanni adopts to manage his own suffering, which is to hastily pack a suitcase and leave immediately after an argument. He ignores phone calls and messages for two or three days, leaving Beatrice to suffer the anguish of not knowing whether he is alive or dead or his whereabouts.

The concrete issues keeping them apart are fairly commonplace and for the most part disagreements over how to raise their younger son. However, the reaction is disproportionate; as if a sudden gust of wind fills the sails of Giovanni's ship and in no time at all he is beyond reach. An adverse turn of events decided by envious gods or in today's language, could Giovanni be the symptom-bearer of a transgenerational unconscious mandate?[4]

He always returns home after a few days and despite repeated promises that it will not happen again, the behaviour has continued and even escalated.

Beatrice eventually responds to her husband's actions by asking him for a trial separation; in this way, she too is seeking a distance to protect herself from feelings of despair and abandonment. However, she is keen to find out what he actually does when he disappears. He tells her that he sleeps in his office, works during the day and spends the nights alone, waiting for the feelings of anger and disappointment towards Beatrice to die down. One night, after imagining where Giovanni might have taken refuge, in desperation, Beatrice goes to look for him at his office but gets no answer when she knocks on the door.

The unyielding door triggers fantasies of possible erotic adventures and the untruthfulness of Giovanni's version of events. Then, during another lonely night, plagued by the thought that he might have had a fatal accident, Beatrice telephones all the emergency departments in her area. The fruitless search leaves her with a sense of relief and disappointment that the epilogue does not end with Giovanni's death, perhaps unconsciously desired.

After a few meetings in which they both talk a great deal about their present difficulties, their accounts become interspersed with flashbacks that help reconstruct their history as individuals and as a couple.

It was precisely this aspect of the couple's narrative structure that led me to make a first association with the *Odyssey*, an ancient text in which the narrative departs from the chronology of events. This characteristic only comes to life in Book VI-VII when Odysseus, having left Calypso's Island, reaches the land of the Phaeacians, where he meets Nausica. Here, Odysseus, once admitted to the court of King Alcinous, begins to recount the events preceding his arrival, an extended flashback through which the reader learns of the many adventures and misadventures Odysseus experienced during his 20-year absence from Ithaca.

In addition to the content of adventure, Homer's narrative strategy of alternation between flashback (analexis) and flashforward (prolexis) makes the *Odyssey* an engaging tale. The epic poem about Odysseus's return to Ithaca constitutes the archetype of the modern adventure novel and the matrix of every theory of storytelling.[5] Initially, the switching back and forth between Giovanni's and Beatrice's accounts and their ability to oscillate between memories and desires for the future produces several effects. The first of these is my identification with their experience: a feeling of wanting to understand and yet wanting to distance myself when their exchange escalates to a shouting match of the deaf.

The account of their meeting and the important stages of their relationship through flashbacks evokes a new awareness of how text and weaving (*testo* and *tessitura*), which share a common etymology in Italian, led to the first association with Penelope's shroud and the tale of Odysseus.

Moreover, once these two characters have entered the field through my uncommunicated association, I begin to reflect on the many traits they appear to have in common with Giovanni and Beatrice, for example, Beatrice's wavering about whether to attempt to rebuild the relationship or seek divorce, Giovanni's fleeing behaviour that is untempered by the responsibility of having children – their fantasies of fortuitous landings on islands of Eden-like happiness.

Lastly, the tears that so often accompany Beatrice's efforts to put experiences and feelings into words reminds me that the very act of telling and retelling involves a painful return home as she retraces memories of moments full of happiness and harmony, but from which she feels irretrievably distanced by their being in the past. By contrast, her wish to divorce holds the lure of landing on the island of the Lotus-Eaters where everything from the past is forgotten. Initially, talking to each other in therapy represents the couple's only point of contact, the starting point from which to find a tolerable level of closeness after many disadventures.

Calypso: a trial love affair

As mentioned earlier, I try to describe my work with Giovanni and Beatrice as a sort of prototype of the couple relationship and then revisit select episodes from the *Odyssey* from the perspective of a relationship between a man and a woman.

Giovanni: Before Beatrice (my wife), I had only had one real long-term relationship with a girl from high school. At the beginning, it was Beatrice who fell in love with me. I was not looking for a girlfriend, I let myself be carried along by her feelings, and it was nice for a while. I felt special in the group because my friends would ask me what it was like to be with a girl and what we did together, and they were very curious about what she looked like when she was naked because she was really beautiful.

But then she used to get jealous, she would ask to see me every day, and if I went out with my friends without inviting her, she would sulk for days. By the time I started university, I was starting to feel suffocated and we were arguing nonstop to the point that even Beatrice agreed that it would be better if we went our separate ways. However, after those first months when I didn't know how to behave, I did love her very much and I don't think there will ever be a time like that again.

Giovanni, like Odysseus, tells of a time on a happy island after drifting there by chance following a shipwreck. On the island of Ogygia, Odysseus meets the beautiful nymph Calypso who soon falls in love with him. Odysseus eventually comes to share her affections. The Greek etymology of Calypso alludes to hiding, and it is precisely in this isolation and exclusion from the world that Odysseus finds solace and care. However, this feeling of fulfilment would soon give way to feelings of suffocation and homesickness.

So for both genders, there is almost always a trial period in couple relationships, hidden from the watchful eyes of parents and disconnected from relationships with peer groups.

It is short-lasting and inhabited by the illusion of the immortality of the feelings, the dazzling beauty of the youthful, vigorous bodies, and fantasies that colour the perception of every first gesture.

When Giovanni, like Odysseus, alighted on the shores of the island, he was feeling somewhat battle-worn after conflict with his parents. Even experiences with his peers and his first attempts to stand out as an individual had depleted him psychically.

Initially the discovery of love feels to Giovanni like landing in a sort of new maternal womb, and a new state of symbiosis that replaces the recently resolved symbiosis with his mother. Isolation gives the couple a sense of fulfilment and peace until the feeling loses some of its intensity and being isolated from the group starts to feel suffocating. The longing to return home sometimes coincides with a longing to regain independence by breaking free from an excessive dependence.

Calipso: Son of Laertes, sprung from Zeus, Odysseus of many devices, would'st thou then fare now forthwith home to thy dear native land! Yet, even so fare thee well. Howbeit if in thy heart thou knewest all the measure of woe it is thy fate to fulfil before thou comest to thy native land thou wouldest abide here and keep this house with me, and wouldest be immortal, for all thy desire to see thy wife for whom thou longest day by day. Surely not inferior to her do I declare myself to be either in form or stature, for in no wise is it seemly that mortal women should vie with immortals in form or comeliness.[6] (*Odyssey* Book V, vv 203–224)

Then Odysseus of many wiles answered her, and said:

Odisseo: Mighty goddess, be not wroth with me for this. I know full well of
myself that wise Penelope is meaner to look upon than thou in comeliness and in stature, for she is a mortal, while thou art immortal and age-
less. But even so I wish and long day by day to reach my home, and to
see the day of my return. (*Odyssey* Book V, vv 224–227)

The relationship matures, like all couple relationships do after weathering pain
and hardship, but there is still a striving for the feeling of being at home and striking the right balance between fusion and separateness.

Circe: the encounter with Eros

Circe lives on the island of Aeaea in a palace guarded by ferocious beasts. She
bewitches Odysseus's men with her voice and poisonous potions, and then turns
them into pigs. She attempts to do the same to Odysseus, but above all she is driven
by her desire to have a sexual encounter with him.

Circe: Surely thou art Odysseus, the man of ready device, who Argeiphontes
of the golden wand ever said to me would come hither on his way home
from Troy with his swift, black ship. Nay, come, put up thy sword in its
sheath, and let us two then go up into my bed, that couched together in
love we may put trust in each other.

Odysseus: Circe, how canst thou bid me be gentle to thee, who hast turned my
comrades into swine in thy halls, and now keepest me here, and with
guileful purpose biddest me go to thy chamber, and go up into thy bed,
that when thou hast me stripped thou mayest render me a weakling and
unmanned? Nay, verily, it is not I that shall be fain to go up into thy
bed, unless thou, goddess, wilt consent to swear a mighty oath that thou
wilt not plot against me any fresh mischief to my hurt.

So I spoke, and she straightway swore the oath to do me no harm, as
I bade her. But when she had sworn, and made an end of the oath, then
I went up to the beautiful bed of Circe. (*Odyssey* Book X, vv 330–335,
335–347)

Odysseus too is driven by the same desire, as becomes apparent when he defines
Circe's bed and the encounter that has yet to be experienced as beautiful.

So Circe can be seen both as a character and as an emblem of the erotic enchant-
ment that sparks and accompanies every experience of falling in love. All reason,
prudence and consideration of propriety are cast into oblivion – an intoxicating and
potentially deadly poison. Odysseus lands on this island whose name derives from
the Greek word for dawn (Eos) and soon becomes Circe's lover. He secures his

companions' release from Circe's spell and then spends a full year with her, while banishing his longing to return to Ithaca from his heart.

In the therapy room: a conversation with many multiple echoes of similarity.

Beatrice: Sure, at the beginning, it was very different from now: he wanted to be with me all the time as if he had to explore and get to know me. For Giovanni, I was like a wild, mysterious territory he was intensely attracted to. Our main concern was to find a place where we could make love.

Giovanni: In my eyes, it was as if she were the only woman in the world. I was in my early twenties, and the fact that I could land such a beautiful girl made me think I could achieve anything: a degree, a prestigious job, a satisfying life, travel and success.

Homer recounts how Odysseus climbed up onto a rock and saw a strip of land, unmistakably an island with the sea encircled around it like a garland. Once ashore, they come to Circe's dwelling in a clearing in the centre of the island. All around, Odysseus adds, one could see wide roads.

If we consider this landscape as the transformation of an experience into a dreamlike image, we could say then that the perception of the loved one's uniqueness and centrality is a universal characteristic of falling in love. A clearing in the heart of a happy island from which, in the imagination, wide roads stretch away.

And yet the first disillusions are soon to arrive.

The turning of his companions into pigs injects something crude and repulsive into the tale.

Something foreseen by intuition but promptly expunged from consciousness by primordial instinct to which the animality of the pigs refers.

Odysseus: Thence we sailed on, grieved at heart, glad to have escaped death, though we had lost our dear comrades; and we came to the isle of Aeaea, where dwelt fair-haired Circe, a dread goddess of human speech, own sister to Aetes of baneful mind. (*Odyssey* Book X, vv 132–137)

Circe's unruly mane of hair acts as a counterpoint to the sweetness of the singing. An aesthetic detail that alludes to a lack of docility and composure juxtaposed with the sweetness of the words and messages that accompany the experience of falling in love.

Beatrice: At the beginning, he used to write me lovely messages and tell me that our relationship would last forever. When I think back to that first year, I can remember being disappointed by the way he acted at times; I was sorry to give up what I wanted. Sometimes I found him a bit stiff, but they were fleeting thoughts that soon got brushed aside whenever we had sex.

Perhaps the ferocious beasts that defend the island of falling in love and dawning of love, bite and chase away any rational thoughts or insights into the true nature of the other. They banish any intrusive thought that might permeate the intoxicating discovery of Eros.

And still the couple soon face a gradual process of disillusionment: otherness makes itself felt in hitherto unshared everyday gestures. A defensive solution to the pain of the other's diversity is sought through quietly acquiescing to their distancing.

The sirens

The island of the Sirens was stony and barren. Its rocky shores were littered with the corpses of their victims, a bleak and macabre landscape that contrasted with its strange dwellers' enchanting song.

Sirens: Come hither, as thou farest, renowned Odysseus, great glory of the Achaeans; stay thy ship that thou mayest listen to the voice of us two. For never yet has any man rowed past this isle in his black ship until he has heard the sweet voice from our lips. Nay, he has joy of it, and goes his way a wiser man. For we know all the toils that in wide Troy the Argives and Trojans endured through the will of the gods, and we know all things that come to pass upon the fruitful earth. (Book 12, vv 181–191)

There is something rocky and barren in Giovanni and Beatrice's life as a couple that is overlaid by an irrepressible desire to hear the other sing their praises and acknowledge their worth.

Giovanni: I'm not in a good place; I feel depressed. I've wanted to tell you this for a long time, but I've been finding myself looking at other women with interest. I avoid spending time with colleagues with whom I might be tempted to have a fling. You are the best wife I could ever wish for, but I feel bad.

Beatrice: (stops crying) I believe that losing your prestigious job has profoundly changed you, and now you just look for exciting moments that make you feel like a god again.

Her interpretation is striking and very pertinent, as if she knows that it is not only other women's bodies that attract her husband.

Giovanni is visibly struck; he denies it but at the same connects with the undeniable emotional truth of her words.

The sirens' terrible power, prototype of temptation, lies precisely in their ability to speak to each man differently, unearthing their most secret and strongest desires and using them as temptation.

The sirens promise Odysseus the celebration of his heroic past and knowledge of all worldly things.

Having a new partner would allow Giovanni, like Odysseus, to retell his whole story and win another woman's passionate admiration. However, the risk of mirroring a false-self in his own story is nothing but a way to lose himself in the eternal return of the same, interrupting the journey towards the future.

It is only by knowing these weaknesses of his soul that Odysseus is able to save himself. Similarly in the case of this couple, being able to put their feelings and experiences into words with sincerity and gaining an increasing awareness of their own and each other's selfish and dependent needs may help avert shipwreck.

However, after getting past the island of the Sirens, Odysseus has to sail through the treacherous Straits of Messina, inhabited by two sea monsters: Scylla and Charybdis.

Transposed to the vicissitudes of a couple, we could say that overcoming a crisis is no guarantee of danger-free navigation. If it is indeed true that overcoming adversity restores a sense of capability, it is also true that it brings about a sense of loss of the relationship's previous integrity or wholeness.

After Odysseus has survived the seduction of the Sirens, Homer describes how he saves himself from a whirlpool created by Scylla by clinging to the roots of a fig tree while six of his best rowers perish in the shipwreck. He loses these men because it seems dishonourable to him that they should wear weapons without using them and entrusts their safety to prayers to Crataide, the monster's sea goddess mother.

Wearing weapons only for the purpose of defence and renouncing the use of attack is also a challenge in relationships, especially when navigating turbulent waters.

Nausica: arriving at integration

Following Giovanni's declaration of his sexual desire for other women and the unveiling of the underlying vulnerabilities, the couple in therapy experiences another crisis. Giovanni, in particular, feels hurt and forced to rethink what drove him to give up his previous managerial position for private practice in an area of lesser social prestige.

The malaise that could have driven him to seek out new adventures mutates itself into a more intense feeling of a depressive nature but may also be a harbinger of possible future transformation.

The age-old relationship with his father, who had picked out his brother as the son capable of social success, returns with a vengeance. Giving up the prestigious job may have been an attempt to withdraw from a losing battle, on both concrete and affective levels. A powerful storm ensues, also in Giovanni's heart; the hunger for affection makes itself felt but cannot find a landing place.

The immersion in this icy water lasts several weeks until Giovanni, like Odysseus, is washed up on a patch of dry land, stripped of the clothes that had shielded him and covered with encrustations of salt that stung his open wounds.

Odysseus's arrival on the island of the Phaeacians marks the end of the wrath of Neptune who had wrecked his ships many times to avenge the blinding of Polyphemus, his son. Something similar happens when Giovanni is able to elaborate, at least partially, his age-old anger towards his father for making him feel second-born and second-best regardless.

After this last stage of a 20-year journey, Odysseus can return to Ithaca. Giovanni emerges from the shipwreck with an old yet also new desire: to be home.

Giovanni: I want to stop leaving home as I have been doing. I want to be with you and the children. Over the last days, I've been thinking back to when I saw you for the first time. Being younger, I had the impression that you were repelled and a bit afraid of me but also that you were attracted to my body.

Beatrice: That's the way it was. You were also very seductive with words. But anyway, it is useless for you to try to walk down the same road again, remembering the beginning and hoping that it will make me go back to being a blank page to write on.

Much like in the fourth book of the *Odyssey*, when Odysseus meets Nausica, Giovanni is the wounded hero, and Beatrice is the young woman who although hopeful of finding love is not willing to let herself be ravaged by a stranger. She is brave and cautious.

In their narrative, besides the inevitable idealisation of the other, there is an emergent capacity to grasp the difficulty of meeting with the other not only through the body but also through the mind.

As seductive aspects of their early relationship, they mention both physical attraction and harmony achieved by communicating through words. In the description of these early stages, they both speak of the potential risk inherent in losing oneself in the experience of being accepted, in the experience of genuine moments of meeting. Privitera, in his book commenting on the *Odyssey*, wrote that a war veteran can lose the chance of returning not only by being killed but also by being seduced and waylaid by the hospitality of those who welcome him along the way.

Like Odysseus, Beatrice knows that retracing her steps cannot transform her into a blank page. Remaining in a long-past place means interrupting the circularity of the journey: the return to Ithaca, the return to the difficulty of meeting after such a long absence.

Penelope: the old and new companion

Penelope re-encounters Odysseus but does not recognise him, disillusioned and frustrated as she is by the many times she entertained the hope of his return.

The ruse of the cloth, woven by day and unravelled by night, can also be seen as the arduous internal process of building up hope alternated with its collapse. Something similar can be observed in the way Odysseus's journey is traversed by the red thread of his longing for Ithaca and by the many adventures that temporarily erase it.

Odysseus returns to Penelope's life when she is, in all likelihood, a mature woman whose interest in sexuality has waned due to age and being no longer used to using her body to create an experience of intimacy. Penelope does not recognise Odysseus because she is also struggling to recognise herself in this old and new role of wife. And yet it is no coincidence that they reconnect through what they share most intimately, the secret construction of their marital bed. Timewise, this mutual recognition occurs after Odysseus has slain all of the suitors with Penelope's unwitting involvement.

From a psychic perspective, in this arbitrary reinterpretation of Homer's tale, the *Proci*, or pretenders to the throne, can be considered a symbol of all the experiences that have threatened the couple. Therefore, restoring its unity entails being able to purge oneself from the temptations, the grudges and the many disappointments that have extinguished desire.

This is a bloody and brutal operation insofar as it also entails a partial amputation of the self. Yet in order to remain in the here and now and rediscover sexual intimacy, the mind needs to make a clean sweep of the past and stem the onslaught of painful memories, not by erasing them but by using a newly acquired ability to keep them in the background.

Penelope succeeds in recognising Odysseus after the nurse discovers his true identity, which Odysseus compels her to keep secret.

There is then no direct help through words but an ability to draw indirectly from another woman's experience.

Beatrice: I felt something had changed inside me. When he came home, I told myself that there would be yet another disappointment, but then I remembered a conversation with a much older friend of mine who had been separated for many years. Whilst talking about my current difficulties, she confided that she regretted her own separation and regretted not pursuing the option of living together relatively separately under the same roof. The solution of living under a façade doesn't feel right to me: either we are a couple, or we go our separate ways. But I also thought that a partial separation would be right in the sense of avoiding getting lost in excessive expectations.

Penelope chooses not to wait any longer and holds a contest that will choose her new spouse. She thus enacts her hatred of the abandonment which for so many years she has kept at bay: a form of vengeance. In Ithaca, Odysseus carries out a massacre before making himself known to his wife.

Therefore, after the narration of heroic deeds and trials, the epilogue unveils the undercurrent of rage which accompanied both Penelope and Odysseus.

Repeatedly, Homer describes Odysseus as a gallant warrior, brave in battle and capable of great cunning and shrewdness.

In Greek, however, his name has an entirely different meaning. It derives from the verb >οδ'υσσομαι meaning to hate, to be hated and also to be bad-tempered. Throughout the book it is difficult to grasp this aspect lying hidden within the etymology of the name, until it emerges in the epilogue.

The *Odyssey* recounts events that take place after the end of the Trojan War but returns to a war-like scenario in its finale. However, it is a private war in which there are no winners or losers, almost as if to suggest that while conflict often runs like a thread through the relationship, its composition is capable of weaving the fabric of the existential journey of every individual and couple.

Notes

1 Dodd wrote " My main concern is not with the dream-experience of the Greeks, but with the Greek attitude to dream experience". Odyssey could be read like "dreams closely related to myth, of which it has been well said that it is the dream-thinking of the people, as the dream is the myth of the individual". (Dodds 1951, p.103) See also Dodds 2009.
2 Calvino published this thoughts first on the italian newspaper La Repubblica in 1981. "It will always be 'Odyssey'" was the title of the article in which Italo Calvino presented the first volume of the Valla-Mondadori edition of Odyssey. Now in Calvino 2001.
3 Placanica 1993; Malerba 1997.
4 Kaës 1993.
5 Italo Calvino sustained this hypothesis in the preface of Privitera's book (2005).
6 All the citations of the *Odyssey* are taken from *The Odyssey, English Translation by A. T. Murray, PH.D.*, Harvard University Press/William Heinemann, Ltd., 1919.

Chapter 6

Color field painting
Bion[1] and Rothko[2]

Paraphrasing Rothko's sentence, "A painting is not a picture of an experience, it is an experience"[3] we might say that there are times when a seminar is the sharing of an experience and an experience in itself. A journey that may bring into view something "that has always been there but we have never seen it that way". Author Jan Brokken describes this experience during his train trip to Daugavpils, the birth-place of Mark Rothko:

> Two colours dominate outside the window: the red of the sky and the green of the woods. The red is bright, streaked with lighter and more uncertain shades; the green is interrupted by the black and brown of the branches. These are sur-faces that I see, surfaces at the top and the bottom, contrasts that need each other: the sky only becomes sky when there is earth, the red becomes redder thanks to the darker lower band. A painting flows out of the window: a picture that never ends, intense and disturbing, quiet and deep as Rothko's painting. Painters show us what has always been there, but we have never seen it that way.
> (Brokken 2010, pp. 388–389)

Reading the transcript of Bion's seminar in Paris in 1978 is a journey in which one re-encounters so many of the theoretical insights he explored in his writings that there is a sensation of blurring; it is almost like looking out of a train window. However, staying attuned to the emotions evoked and attempting to capture the imagery as it springs to mind helps to avoid being overwhelmed by this sensa-tion, by what is known and yet unknown, and one begins to glimpse relational landscapes from an unprecedented point of view. My own reading experience was repeatedly associated with images of paintings: as illustrations of the con-cepts and pictograms of the emotions evoked by the dialogue between Bion and the audience.

This chapter is a personal response to Bion's aesthetic conceptions and an attempt to make explicit the parallels between his theories and Marc Rothko's works. Bion and Rothko focused on the emotional experience at the heart of their work and the tension towards the truth.[4] Moreover, the originality of both of these men, who were almost contemporaries, even if from different places and with different life

DOI: 10.4324/9781003388838-7

experiences, is rooted in a particular way of understanding representation. Both were interested in technique as a means to produce a specific effect, that of allowing those who come across their work to immerse themselves in the analytic experience in Bion's case and the artistic experience in Rothko's.

To achieve this effect, Rothko changed his means of expression, using elaborate methods bordering on alchemy, and took almost obsessive care of the exhibition design of his works.

In the trilogy *Memory of the Future*, Bion used dreams and dreaming and the theatre to express his ideas. Both Bion and Rothko thus developed an innovative technique to achieve an experience-evoking representation, a method not fully appreciated until long after their deaths.

Although Bion's seminar in Paris style is more discursive and therefore seemingly more accessible than *Memory of the Future*, it has a structure in which ideas are presented in a non-rhetorical way, removed from the classic form of a seminar. Nevertheless, it is a form that bears some resemblance to unorthodox landscape composition in figurative art.

Even though the two research methods are very different, Bion and Rothko assume that a work of art can only exist if an interlocutor is willing to meet it and feel emotions. In the Paris seminar, Bion's interest focuses on the psychoanalytic and artistic processes and stresses the relationship between the two disciplines. He arrived to say that if an analyst did not consider himself an artist, he was in the wrong profession. Bion, therefore, sets out to encourage the audience and reader to discover their artistic inclinations. But why should a psychoanalyst venture into the field of another discipline? Would he not risk losing his own identity and specificity? What is the use of being an artist in the therapeutic relationship with a patient?[5]

One possible answer lies in Bion's interest in the "inaccessible part of the mind"[6] and the psychotic part of the personality as is testified by his return to these themes at the Paris seminar. Bion's early work as a psychiatrist focused on psychotic phenomena in the group, and the psychotic part of personality remained one of his research interests for his whole life. To gain access and study them, the analyst has to take on the patient's pathology, something that Bion himself did not advocate, or become capable of making fuller use of a creative and imaginative area of the mind and tune in on sensory levels. The artistic and psychoanalytic processes converge precisely in the endeavour to tune into emotional and sensory experiences.

However, one area of divergence is that the process of artistic expression appears to be more geared towards emotional expression and sharing at a distance. Instead, psychoanalysis challenges achieving emotional unison and focuses on transforming painful emotions in the here and now of the encounter.[7]

Moreover, confronting Bion's Paris seminar and Rothko's last exhibition makes it possible (although not always true) to think that psychoanalysis can offer the mind more tools – thoughts helpful to escape from the nameless terror of death: both when it presents itself in "madness" and when it becomes an experience at the end of life.[8,9]

Last public offerings and viewpoints

As mentioned, the chapel in Houston was home to the last exhibition of Rothko's works, meticulously curated by himself, especially about the interaction between colour and light reflected on the canvases. Specifically, Rothko exhibited 14 predominantly black and grey canvases to give the viewer an immersive experience of his work. The strategies Rothko intentionally applied. He believed that colour, aided by light, could enter into a relationship with the soul, generating a surprisingly emotional experience.

In a similar vein, Bion's expository style in his Paris seminar (and in his writings in general) gives his audience and readership access to an entirely new vantage point and renders the presentation of ideas and experience more emotional than cognitive. On a first reading, the emotional response may be a mix of attraction and repulsion.

We might wonder why Bion chose to address so many issues in the relatively short timeframe of a seminar.

Why are we drawn in by the breadth of a discourse as vast as a large canvas?

We may gain some insight by reading Rothko's reflections on the space within the painting and the relationship between the painting and the wall. When asked about the monumental size of his works, Rothko wrote:

> I paint very large pictures . . . precisely because I want to be intimate and human. To paint a small picture is to place yourself outside your experience, to look upon an experience as a stereopticon view or with a reducing glass. However, you paint the larger picture; you are in it.
>
> (Rothko 2006)

Therefore, the size of a canvas and embedding theoretical concepts within such a wide range of psychoanalytic issues during a conference may evoke an experience of inclusion. Amongst the wide range of issues, we may recognise a personal reflection linked to one of our own experiences. The sheer breadth of the Paris seminar's content gives us the feeling of being in the audience and participating in collective thinking.

Another formal aspect contributing to the feeling of inclusion is the offering of different concepts in close succession. This expository style creates a very different experience from the one we might have when a speaker presents the arguments for his ideas in a logical sequence. This method of exposition, which may seem on the surface to be characterised by haphazard free association, belies a creative process that may perhaps be made more explicit by some of Rothko's aesthetic considerations.

On the occasion of the Fifteen Americans show in 1952, Dorothy Miller recalled that Rothko

> wanted to have the four walls of the gallery completely covered with paintings touching one another. He did not wish to accept the Museum gallery's lighting,

proposing instead to have blazing lights in the centre of the ceiling. Rothko . . . wanted to surround and saturate viewers with his large, vibrant paintings as if to give museum visitors no choice but to look at them.

(Breslin 1993, p. 303)

However, alongside the experience of inclusion created by the particular expository style, the reader of Bion's Paris seminar may also experience a rather unpleasant feeling that has to do with the opposite of immersion or being at the heart of the experience. We might envisage a root of this feeling of distance in the observation that Bion rarely gives direct answers to the audience's questions. Thus, even if we are interested in what is being said or read, there is an experience of not being on the same page.

Bion makes this clearer by likening this experience to the analytic encounter with the patient:

There are two people in the room who come together at the same time, in the same place, but the directions in which they are thinking are different.

(Bion 2014)

As well as being aware of this phenomenon in the analytic couple, Bion seems to be conscious of it in the encounter with his listening audience. He begins the lecture by explaining that he will use English and not the French he learnt at school for reasons that will become apparent. The reasons may be guessed at, perhaps understood, starting from the experience of an irrevocable distance involving the language.

I would like you to regard this as a working conference where this problem faces all of us.

And a little later:

So, listening to the conversation between yourself and your patient, what language is being talked, either by him or her, or yourself or both of you.

(Bion 2014)

There is a thin line between people, individuals and groups regardless of whether or not they speak the same language. Even as they reach out to understand something of the other, as occurs during the analytic encounter or at a conference. It is important for the psychoanalyst to be aware of this distance and to learn how to deal with it.

Bion, like Rothko, was well aware of the profound emotional experiences a psychoanalyst (or painter) would go through. For example, they know how emotional contact could evoke a satisfying feeling of unity or frustration:

I am interested only in expressing basic human emotions . . . and the fact that lots of people break down and cry when confronted with my pictures shows that I can communicate those basic human emotions.

(Rothko 1957)

However, the gulf between this intimate self-exposure and his disappointment at not being appreciated would lead Rothko to experience an inner turmoil that he tried to ward off or manage by assuming an ideologically opposed position towards his clients.

For Rothko, the gulf between his idiom and the public became a source of repeated deep disappointment and conflict rather than a starting point to move towards thought, as it would be in the analytic encounter.

The leap from figurative to abstract

Bion said something about how to leap out from reality on the analytic encounter from the first lines of the seminar. If he were a painter, we could say that he passed from figurative to abstract.

Rothko did the same: he took the centrality of emotion to the extreme, expanding the chromatic mantle until it overpowered every figure.[10,11] There is no symbolic representation, perspective and title in Rothko's mature paintings. There is no story.

After having shared the problem of linguistic distance with the audience, Bion offers a first analytic example of how he adopts a non-realistic, non-historical attitude.

He presents to the audience a patient who complains about unsatisfactory family life. It would be classic telling but not for the following: "I am unsure what family he is talking about" (Bion 2014).

We are taken aback and then, as we digest the surprise that has shattered the obvious, an emotional movement of reconciliation begins to form. We may find ourselves agreeing with Bion's statement because many families create dissatisfaction; belonging to a group, be it large or small, is always tricky.

However, Bion further undermines the sense of familiarity we have when we think that what we see is what exists:

> [A] young man of twenty-five complains of having an unsatisfactory family life.... I ask him his age, and he says forty-two. Forty-two? But I said twenty-five just now. As I see him more closely, I notice lines on his face, and every now and then, I think he looks more like sixty-two than forty-two or twenty- five. Well, what is his age?
>
> (Bion 2014)

Our senses dictate the idea that something exists; placing it in a spatiotemporal framework is an arbitrary conjecture. It is a point of view. If others exist only according to the schemas of our mind – as Bion seems to suggest – and if we look at them by placing them in a temporal space defined by perception and cognition, we end up seeing only what we already know. Therefore, age and the conjectures that may arise from it are irrelevant to an analytic encounter.

Something like the possible murmur of the audience resonates in the reader. So this premise will end up dragging everything and everyone towards a nihilistic wilderness. How can such an indisputable detail like a patient's age or the fact that the family he is talking about is his family become irrelevant in one fell swoop?

Bion urges the audience to move from content to emotions in a few lines. What Bion is doing is the same Rothko did in the 1950s when he abandoned figurative art to express his feelings only through shapes and colours[12]:

> The familiar identity of things has to be pulverised to destroy the infinite associations with which our society increasingly enshrouds every aspect of our environment.
>
> (Rothko 2006, p. 59)

and again,

> The progression of a painter's work, as it travels in time from point to point, will be toward clarity: toward the elimination of all obstacles between the painter and the idea and between the idea and the observer. As examples of such obstacles, I give (among others) memory, history and geometry, which are swamps of generalization from which one may pull out parodies of ideas (which are ghosts) but never an idea in itself. To achieve this clarity is, inevitably, to be understood.
>
> (Rothko 2006, p. 65)

Considering memory, history and geometry as obstacles echoes Bion's saying that a psychoanalyst should listen to his patient without memory and desire. This effort allows him to attune himself as far as possible to the emotional content of what is being communicated and speak to the patient with words that do not explain the emotion but allow him to experience and understand it. The analyst's language comes from their experience of emotion, an effective way of speaking that comes closer to creating an image than a speech. Bion writes:

> A painter, for example, may believe that a painting should be true to truth, should show you some aspect of reality which you might otherwise not notice.
>
>   It is certainly not somebody who can deceive your eyes to make you think that there is a tree there when there isn't one, but somebody who has made you see there really is a tree there and its roots even if they are underground.
>
> (Bion 2014)

Bion's patient is no longer a person with a life history, and he is like a spectrum of emotions meeting another range of emotions (those of the analyst). Real life remains outside, barely visible in the outer perimeter of the frame and the setting.

In other words, although it remains in a certain sense excluded, real life is the background from which the facts of the analysis emerge; in the foreground of the setting is the emotional experience created by the infinite shades of the colours as they come to face each other.

Rothko writes:

> I think of my picture as dramas; the shapes in the pictures are the performers. They have been created from the need for a group of actors who are able to

move dramatically without embarrassment and execute gestures without shame. Neither the action nor the actors can be anticipated or described in advance. They begin as an unknown adventure in an unknown space.

(2006, p. 58)

The new conception of space: do you believe we can choose the vertex?

Starting from this operation of abstraction from reality, of focusing on emotions and of a new relationship between what is in the foreground and background, both Bion and Rothko came to transform actual events into emotional narratives, people into characters. Also, *space as the physiological basis of a painting*[13] or setting as the frame of a session became something new.

Rothko writes:

If, for example, I were to undertake the discussion of "space", I would first have to disabuse the word from its current meanings. I would have to redefine and distort it.

(2006, p. 92)

If we did not know its author, we might assume Bion had written this sentence.

Instead of making the setting and relational space an ingredient of analysis, Bion strove to reorient its complexity. He went beyond the concepts of external or internal space, relational space and setting, and introduced the idea of space as an experience.

In a psychoanalytic experience, it is impossible to separate the two subjects by defining the observer and the observed; there may be multiple perspectives, and whatever material appears has many facets.

Choosing what to observe extends a focus centred exclusively on the patient to include the observer, and the depth of experience determines what we see, "and the more you know about yourself, the more you know which vertex to choose in order to look at the problem" (Bion 2014).

Rothko did much the same thing in his painting when he broke from the classic relationship between image and wall while painting on traditional, mostly rectangular canvases. Rothko transformed the wall from an external space and mere support for the canvas into a plastic element within the same experience the painting wishes to evoke. He transformed the picture into a wall incorporating the external space and subverting the in and out experience; there is no distance between the work and the real world. He made pictorial space into an area of experience in which the boundaries were not immediately defined, opening up new vistas of observation.

The complex relationship between colours and people

While the audience of the Paris seminar and the reader is still immersed in an unsettling experience, busy digesting the transformation of a clinical history into a dreamlike adventure, Bion complicates matters further by proposing another question. Referring again to the patient who may have different ages depending on the vertex from which one looks at him, he asks his listeners (and readers) to decide whether they would be willing to take on such a patient. Again, he does not refer to diagnostic criteria but invites them to tune into the emotions experienced by the analyst and the patient and those invoked by reading a book, listening to a piece of music, or seeing a painting. He then encourages the audience to give shape to their emotional response by asking: how would you describe your feeling of an engagement or lack of it through a colour, a piece of music, a story?

Bion then asks his audience to think of a colour to begin the process of transforming the first sensorial impressions evoked by this hypothetical patient into symbolic form, of which colour may be the first step.

He urges the audience to think along the same lines as they should do in analysis.

But no one goes to a seminar expecting to listen more to himself than to the speaker; a participant wishes to take notes on what the presenter says to understand it better and gain some new ideas or technical suggestions. No one predisposes himself to be immersed in a sensory and emotional experience.

If the speaker tells you:

> [G]et out your colours; don't write notes on this story, make marks on the paper. Use a few simple colours like blue, black, yellow, green. Then look at it; you will get an idea of how that patient struck you.
>
> (Bion 2014)

At the very least, you will feel disconcerted and find yourself at a cross-roads: either you walk away shocked, or you take the plunge into a new way of seeing.

Bion proposes a re-evaluation of the imperceptible shapeless sensations, thoughts and emotions that present themselves to the mind without meaning. This sprinkle of microscopic, intermittent, disordered fragments, scattered in an undefined mental space amongst unorganised ideas, gives rise to something still formless, orderless that has neither a before nor an after. Yet, amid this disturbing chaos, it is precisely here that the seed of a developing thought may take root, provided we can cross the barrier of the already known.

Meeting in this sensory realm, at a high emotional temperature, in a place far removed from meaning, is a challenging experience for the psychoanalyst and he has an increased risk of failure.

Similarly, Rothko describes the encounter between picture and onlooker as a *valid marriage of the minds*.[14]

The lack of coupling is grounds for annulment.

Something similar may occur in the analytic encounter when the fear of a leap into unchartered territory produces a response that is a step backwards and not aligned with the other.

Dr Resnik, the organiser of the seminar, tried to enter the heart of the question and immediately after Bion's considerations observes: "It is interesting to note that we say, 'Yellow with envy' in our country, rather than green" (Bion 2014).

Colour is the only connection to what Bion was expounding, and the reader feels nudged in a different direction. Resnik and Bion are not speaking the same language, which reopens the space of experience in the reading. They think and talk differently, and the language with which they attempt to understand each other holds the traces of this difference. In this sense, it is important to stress that Dr Resnik is a famous Argentinean psychoanalyst but, at the same time, a partici- pant faced with what escapes consciousness. His observation reveals retreat in the face of a frightening experience of mental coupling, and this retreat momentarily halts the flow of dialogue.

If this experience were an image, it might be titled *Yellow and Green* as Rothko's 1958 paintings: a block of yellow and a block of green separated by a white line.

Initially, one sees the separation between the two colours in the same way we perceive the distance between Bion's considerations and Resnik's somewhat dys- topian comment.

However, a closer look at the painting or a re-reading of the text reveals a tension towards the encounter. Like patient and analyst, speaker and audience, the reader also feels what it is like to be at the mercy of a new experience, an oscillation between distancing and reaching out to each other.

There are flecks of green in the yellow and lighter areas tending towards yellow in the green. In these subtle overlays of color, one can almost make out a shape: perhaps a door, some windows, a gate, a kind of hallucinosis representing a passage between the inner and outer world. Vision is lost in color, but once amid that non- reality, it return as an immediate need to reconnect with reality.

Rothko's paintings come close to depicting what happens in the analytic dialogue: a sort of pulsation between understanding and distancing, love and hate, desire and fear. In Rothko's *Yellow and Green* painting, there is further suggestion of this experience: the blurry line between the two fields of color. A frayed rope inhabited by a sort of constant tension between coming together and separating. A line aspiring to merge and blend with each of the two colours but instead that remains a white line, different, not assimilable to either yellow or green.

No other painter has visually represented what Bion termed *caesura* as deeply as Rothko:

> Investigate the break; not the analyst, not the analysand; not the unconscious, not the conscious; not sanity, not insanity, but the caesura, the link, the synapse, the (counter) transference, the transitive-intransitive mood.
>
> (Bion 1977, p. 99)

Rothko sometimes painted the caesura between colours as a fracture, a tight black band, intended to represent an obstacle to the relationship between parts of the self or between self and other. In other paintings, such as *Yellow and Green*, he focused more on the relationship between colours. The same can happen in the analytic experience when theories, memories, ideas create mental obstacles to the emotional encounter. Bion paints this experience in words, recounting the moment he became aware of a line separating and unifying the body, being awake or cataleptic:

> I remember a patient who was always very cooperative, and after some time – I fear too long a time – it became clear to me that he was the only patient who did not alter the appearance of the couch; when he left, it was almost as if no one had laid down on it. Then I realized that each time he lay down in the same place. This issue made me think of a kind of catalepsy, of mental catalepsy. I honestly couldn't say that he ever had a dream; I honestly couldn't say that he was awake; he was between these two states. He was not unconscious; he was not conscious. So how did he live in this mental state? Physically he could lie in the same position on the couch: now, it is clear that he was doing the same thing mentally.
>
> (Bion 2014)

To continue the parallel between Rothko and Bion, one can observe that in his definition of *caesura*, Bion describes antithetical fields, but also "the union of the transitive-intransitive mood",[15] the passage from one mental state to another.[16] You are describing a state that facilitates communication to one that hinders it. Here it is as if Bion were looking at a painting where the line that unites and separates is no longer a line; the fields of color themselves delimit a transitional space between one colour and another. A fringed area created by meeting two or more rectangles made up of multiple layers of colour, like the tiny layers of experiences, memories and dreams unique to each person.

Whether represented or described when looking into this area, this frayed line, both analyst and patient and both painter and viewer of the artwork experience anguish and vertigo. At this juncture in which what is mine and what is yours are not definable, one is exposed to a disturbing sense of liquidity.

Bion recommends scrutiny, looking carefully at that which is unclear, not immediately perceptible, immersing one's hands into the words, as though randomly touching scraps of cloth. Using the senses allows us to invent a language that connects and establishes closeness through sharing the same emotional experience.

The catastrophic situation: a concept/an experience

Let us suppose that the search for meaning from the chaos of indecipherable fragments is always at the heart of analytical research, in which case, this proposition becomes the real challenge when probing the unreachable psychotic part of the mind.[17]

Before the question of psychosis is addressed openly and more conceptually in the Paris seminar, something happens which again has to do with the repetition of the experience.

Bion emphasises the necessity of piecing together "bits of what we have been taught, bits of what we have learned, fragments of what the patient has been taught" whilst acknowledging the difficulty in making use of such mental debris.

There is an inaudible and therefore untranscribed comment on psychotic experience from the audience to which Bion replies: "The idea that this is a psychotic experience is very cerebral" (Bion 2014).

What is inaudible? The latent thought in the audience that Bion might be unhinged? Is the inaudible that which cannot be immediately understood?

The audience experiences a state of general disorientation, close to moments of therapeutic impasse.

Bion scrutinises what psychoanalysts have already thought or understood in conceptual terms, along with what does not yet exist and invites us to lean over an edge where the giving up of general rules and methods of analytic understanding creates the feeling of being close to a vacuum of nothingness.

We cannot explore psychosis through the intellect alone, and that is why Bion is proposing not only ideas but also an experience that has the potential to generate new ones. Like Rothko, Bion follows the principle that the artist's task is not to fill the void but to create it.

In other words, Bion arouses feelings of disconcertment in the audience to explore ways of communicating that enable an experience and distinguish those that do not, especially in borderline situations. Bion insists on the difference between science and aesthetic experience, giving almost greater importance to the latter when it comes to penetrating the mysteries of the primitive areas of the mind.

As a researcher, Bion used scientific knowledge, philosophical rigour and the subtle science of logical reasoning. What he is creating in the seminar is a setting where the group can look beyond the darkness, beyond the known threshold.

In this sense, we can compare Bion's Paris seminar to the Rothko Chapel in Houston, the exhibition venue where Rothko designed to display his last 14 grey-black canvases.

The city, a symbolic space of exploration, reminds us of man's unquenchable thirst to discover what lies beyond the earth's confines and our inherent drive to discover what lies beyond the confines of our own experience.

The Rothko Chapel is a windowless octagonal space that deliberately communicates a sense of containment and entrapment at the same time. In this ambiguously intimate space, one can experience the two sides of its confines: if anxiety prevails, one only wishes to get out; if, on the other hand, the intensity of the experience is tolerable, a form of dialogue with the canvases begins; it is something different from what happens in a traditional museum. For example, suppose the eye becomes accustomed to the semi-darkness, and the pervasive blackness calms the sense of disquiet. In that case, nuances begin to emerge; the black rectangles turn grey, the purple ones turn red and change according to the intensity of the natural light coming in through the skylight. The feeling of saturation on being exposed to all that black forces one to concentrate on the weak sunlight filtering through the skylight, which can transform the blackness into a beam of intense darkness.[18]

Something similar may have taken place in Bion's seminar, as can be read between the lines of the last question put to Bion by a member of the audience:

> There are two points I would like to raise. First, here in Paris, there are complaints that there is no discussion about patients' choices. Second, patients want to end the analysis, but their analysts don't want to wean them off.
>
> (Bion 2014)

The question is only partially pertinent to the ongoing discourse, but it lends itself to sharing with the audience that there is no choice for the patient or the speaker. Listening is the only way to get to know better, but listening to content that strays too far from the known produces a sense of claustrophobia and a desire to escape, not dissimilar to when one comes into contact with psychosis and death. Bion seems to grasp this experience, and it is perhaps no coincidence that he ends the seminar with a poem where Death and Beauty, the inexhaustible sources of life, merge.

In their last public expositions, both Bion and Rothko come close to producing a testament to their lives in questioning how great Beauty in avoiding disintegration plays a part.

Bion says in the last lines of the seminar:

> You will have to be able to have the chance of feeling that the interpretation you give is a beautiful one or that you get a lovely response from the patient. This aesthetic element of Beauty makes a complicated situation tolerable.
>
> (Bion 2014)

But, of course, he is referring to the analytic situation.

Still, the mention of Beauty seems to suggest also how he may have been able to get through the many tragic problems he faced during his lifetime. Both Bion and Rothko experienced severe personal setbacks, starting from abandoning their homelands as children.[19] They were men who sought to heal themselves also through aesthetic exploration, leaving us with a rich legacy of invaluable instruments.

The mental wounds caused by severe traumas remain deep within; sometimes they heal, and sometimes they lay dormant for a long time, only to reopen suddenly, as in Rothko's case. The black canvases produced at the end of his life speak of a man who was able to descend to the very depths of the wounds to his soul until it was no longer possible for him to rise again. They tell of the silent scream of a torn existence on the threshold of an ever more unattainable Beauty, of a whole life imagined but never touched.

On the other hand, Bion concludes the seminar with the poem "Vitrail" by José Maria Heredia, an early 19th-century Cuban poet, a choice that brings the reader back in touch with the creative power of the unconscious. In Heredia's poem, which we can find at the end of the seminar transcript, the poet describes the effigies carved on the tombs that cannot hear and with their stone eyes cannot see the colours from the stained-glass window projected onto the floor.

Heredia writes:

[The figures carved on the tombs] look without seeing/the rose of the stained-glass window always in the bud.

(Heredia 1893)

Instead, during the seminar Bion says:

[The carved figures on the tombs] cannot see, cannot hear, but they can see these colours spread out on the floor with their stone eyes.

(Bion 2014)

It is here, in this possibility of seeing where it seems impossible to do so, as in Rothko's black canvases, where there is nothing to see but traces of colour, that the life-giving capacity for creativity resides.

Emotional experience at the core of Bionian psychoanalysis and Rothko paintings

After comparing Bion and Rothko, one might raise questions about the future and the legacy of psychoanalysis. In this last seminar, Bion challenged the convention that words were the only possible expression of ideas. Yet, consistently, at the end of his life, he insisted on the inseparability of words and emotions, proposing to his audience and readers not only ideas but experiences. In the Paris seminar, Bion conveyed his belief that experience must be felt on more than just an intellectual level, and to be therapeutic, it must be felt as "beautiful" – a kind of Beauty born out of the departure from traditional canon that creates space for a new form of existence.

Bionian thought stems from a long critical reflection on traditional psycho-analytic approaches, particularly the Freudian method. The shift is not fueled in opposition to assumptions within Freudian theory but strives for a psychoana-lytic approach that goes beyond the traditional confines. Psychoanalysis, like art, remains an experience that comes close to some kind of truth when it manages to free itself from the rules and restrictions built around it. Sensitive, anamnes-tic, observational data can enter "(the analytic and artistic) discourse as Trojan horses which must be watched most carefully" (as Feyerabend wrote in *Against the Method*), and this could be a starting point for both Bion and Rothko (Feyerabend 1993, p. 60).

Both were freed from the conditioning influences brought to bear by sensory data to propose a search for truth through relationships: the former between people and the latter between rectangular shapes and colours. This is not a historical real-ity, therefore, but a truth embedded in emotion; knowledge springs from emotions and becomes a subjective reflection of the truth through the encounter. Rothko remained faithful to the traditional rectangular-shaped canvas and used a geomet-ric figure and colours used countless times throughout art history. The interaction between shape and background, similarly hued colours that blend only within a thin line that connects them, makes his paintings an experience of freedom and Beauty.

However, to "be fair with Freud" (Derrida 1996), what Bion developed lurked if not in Freud's writings, then in the books he read and in his mind as he refined a different research method for understanding the human mind.

Freud himself probably underlined the following short paragraph about Montaigne in an edition of selected writings:

> Montaigne doesn't know yet what he is capable of, and like all debutants, he imitates. He follows the fashionable, and he follows it even in that which is concerned with ideas.
>
> (Sender 1994, p. 29)

And he was undoubtedly well acquainted with this passage from the Babylonian Talmud:

> Put yourselves into groups to occupy yourselves with the Torah; the Torah can only be acquired in a group. This is according to R. Yosi b. Hanina, for R. Yosi b. R. Hanina, said: How may one explain the verse, "A sword is upon the boasters, and they shall become fools" (Jeremiah 50:36)? So a sword is upon scholars who sit alone to study the Torah. And not only this, but they also become stupid.
>
> (Sender 1994, p. 29)

The two quotations may represent the starting points of Bion's reflections on psychoanalytic theory and method: these sentences focus on his interest in a creative mind, free from the constraints of the known and in the study of group dynamics.

In the Paris seminar, Bion reiterates that at the heart of the psychoanalytic method lies the paradox of a hybrid experience, between narrative representation and imaginative and therefore figurative representation, anticipating criticism for perpetuating the dichotomy between science and art. He reminds us that it is within the thin line where the minds of the analyst and patient merge that new, nuanced ideas may spring to life.

Notes

1 The founder of a psychoanalytic theoretical body called "field theory" transformed speculative academic thinking with the colour of his dreams.

2 The foremost exponent of the Expressionist Color-field Painting movement was the Latvian-born American painter Marcus Rothkowitz, known as Mark Rothko (1903–1970). Clement Greenberg gave the name to this new current of American abstractionism in his essay American-type painting in 1952.

3 As reported by Sophie Tracy, in Breslin (James E. B.) Research Archive on Mark Rothko, box 9, folder 13. See https://www.getty.edu/research/collections/component/10TJC1.

4 Rothko (2006) asserted that the two-dimensionality of canvases destroys the illusion and reveals the truth. "We are for flat forms because they destroy illusion and tell the truth." Letter to Ronald L. 1943 in 35. Also, according to Bion, truth and ultimate reality coincide with "O". "O represents the absolute truth of any object" (Bion 1970, p. 117).

5 Literature is abundant on the relationship between figurative art and psychoanalysis. To mention just a few authors: Segal 1991; Milner 1950; Gedo 1983; Williams 2010; Goldstein 2013.

6 Bion 1957, 1962b, p. 37.

7 "Pictures must be miraculous: the instant one is completed, the intimacy between the creation and the creator is ended". Rothko cited in Ross 1990, p. 1ri.

8 Hartman 2018.

9 I would "like to say to those that think of my pictures as serene – said Rothko – that I have imprisoned the most utter violence in every inch of their surface" (Resin, p. 358) Breslin 1993 p. 355.

10 Rothko 2004.

11 Rothko was aware of the roots of his artwork in the Byzantine era, where the golden background symbolized how divinity prevailed over the figures. Another root was Pierre Bonnard's work. He was a late Impressionist who considered a painting as a series of blobs that link together, forming the object over which parts the eye moves seamlessly.

12 It is not possible to assign a precise date to the beginning of the change of style. However, Melania Mazzucco, in an article in the column "The Museum of the World", published in November 2013, points to the creation of the painting *Violet, Black, Orange, Yellow, White and Red* in 1949.

13 Rothko 2006, p. 97.

14 "The appreciation of art is a true marriage of minds. And in art, as in marriage, lack of consummation is ground for annulment" (Rothko and Gottilieb "Letter to the editor" 1943 in Rothko 2006, p. 35).

15 Bion 1977.

16 Parthenope Bion attributes this meaning to the expression "union of the transitive-intransitive mood" in "Mappe per l'esplorazione psicoanalitica [Maps for psychoanalytic exp.

17 Bergstein 2018.

18 Grotstein 2007.

19 Rootedness is perhaps the most important and most misunderstood requirement of the human soul. It is among the most difficult to define. Through his honest, active and natural participation in the existence of a community that keeps alive, sure treasures of the past and certain presentiments of the future, the human being has a root (Weil 1949, pp. 49–55).

Chapter 7

L'Origine du monde at the end of analysis

Treating a patient obsessed with pornography

As Mr P walked through the anteroom for the first time, in the analyst's mind appeared an image: *Mask of Pain* of Wildt, an early 20th-century sculptor and his self-portrait so entitled (see Figure 7.1).

Once in the consulting room, Mr P sat down and began sobbing. For the next hour, he gave the analyst no room to speak; there was only the sight of the grimaces on this young man's contracted face as he recounted fragments of an obsession with pornography that had taken over his life. The analyst passed him tissues one by one and told him, more through gestures than in words, that she could understand, or better, that perhaps we could try to understand together. The analyst listened and did not feel at all scandalised or judgmental but neither emotionally close.

Used tissues fell to the floor and remained there after the session. The thought of picking them up with bare hands made the analyst feel uncomfortable, and the touching, aversion to the wetness of the bodily fluids, and "disgust" referred to by the man who had just been sitting, involved the analyst more concretely, propelling her towards the first form of sharing.

The analyst looked down at the scrunched-up tissues. How was she to gather them up? The consulting room had to be tidied, and yet she stood there looking at them for some time, paralysed by the absurd feeling of not knowing what to do until she resolved to use a dustpan and broom.

Touching with one's bare hands in psychoanalysis means being able to accommodate the experience of the other, and this is a level of intimate sharing that she had not yet reached with this patient. So, shifting the focus away from the body, she tried to enact a distancing: she hypothesised that the patient's desire for online pornography and compulsive searches for sexual contact with no relation to reality was the outcome of a drama that preceded the symptom. Indeed, this more profound pain would go on to flood the relational field for months, struggling to articulate itself in words.

What is pornography in psychoanalysis?

From which vertex could the analyst listen to tales of secret encounters with countless partners, rich in anatomical detail and palpable excitement?

DOI: 10.4324/9781003388838-8

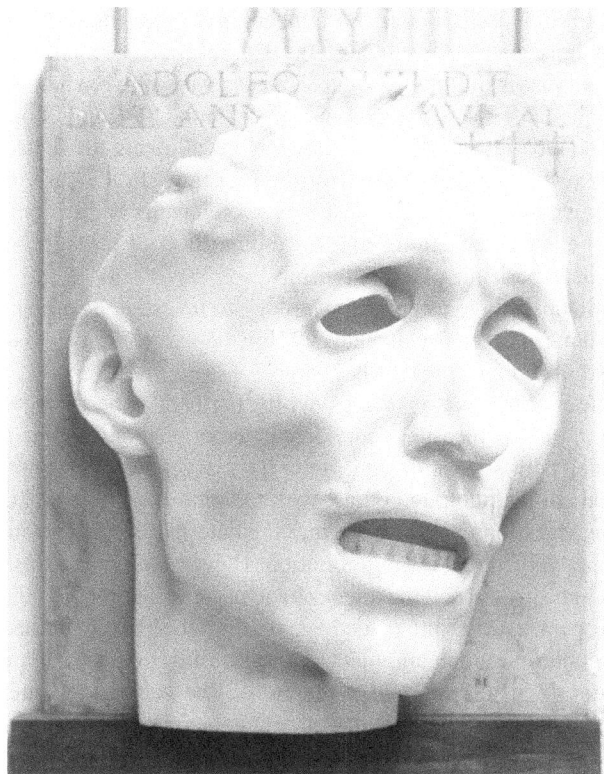

Figure 7.1 A. Wildt, *Mask of Pain.*

First of all, the analyst told herself, it would help to clear the field of all the clichés that an analytical treatment should renounce from the outset. In psychoanalysis, the focal point is not the content or type of symptom.

Taking the post-Bionian developments of the analytic field as a theoretical reference makes it possible, then, to explore which pornographic relationship the patient is actually referring to.

It seems essential to avoid the analytic process becoming an experience devoid of intimate contact between minds and thus an equally pornographic encounter. The first step in this direction could be the provocative hypothesis presented in a small book entitled *Phenomenology and Pornography.*[1]

Its author, Bancalari, argues that phenomenology has radically raised the question of what it means to view pornography, making it a philosophical method that interrogates reality from what reality shows. Thus, both the philosopher and the person obsessed with viewing pornography share a kind of "concupiscence of seeing".

One could argue that there is a substantial difference between a "normal" phenomenon and an obscene act, between observing and interacting with a body and being a spectator of a performance by strangers in an anonymous place. However, the word "concupiscence" helps to close the gap inasmuch as it alludes to a feeling of intense desire that is difficult to control, a passion that overwhelms. In the case of the philosopher, intense desire overwhelms the mind, dragging it out of pushing it beyond the boundaries of what it already knows, allowing it to erase what it has learnt in order to fathom reality as if for the first time. In the case of the person obsessively drawn to internet porn, desire overwhelms the body. It puts the person in search of another body, urging him towards a form of pleasure that excludes thinking and the experience of a relationship.

Is it therefore possible to use phenomenology to investigate pornography, and if so, what does it mean to the psychoanalyst? How do we clear the field of the known in order to start observing from the beginning?

One possible starting point is to consider the perinatal experience, where seeing and moments of intense pleasure coincide with emotional development.

At birth, a newborn's sense of sight is not fully developed and is not the infant's preferred means of maintaining contact with the mother. Before sight, it is touch, proprioceptive sensations and hearing that mediate that sense of continuity with the maternal body occupied during gestation. Babies are born with the ability to perceive light and shadow and the vague shape of figures moving in the immediate space around them. During breastfeeding, on the other hand, the lesser distance enables the infant to fix upon an object whose stability for a certain period allows an initial synthesis of the different perceptions. The baby gazes intensely at the mother's face and at the same time has an oral experience that transforms distress into a pleasant sense of fullness. Thus, the "goodness perceived" is confused with the "goodness seen".[2] The mother's face and body become the privileged form for a satisfying sensation of progressive perceptive synthesis that brings about a new experience of greater emotional fullness.

This last consideration makes it possible to draw some parallels between pornography and primary experience; in erotic play, the early experience of being with the other through the exchange of bodily gestures is re-proposed, a way of seeing and not seeing that is more confused than in everyday life, the possibility of putting aspects of responsibility towards the other into the background is realised, almost as if one could play predatory parts aimed at one's own pleasure.[3]

The hypothesis of a re-actualisation of experiences, paradoxically far removed from genital sexuality, which is instead what characterises pornography, arose from getting to know more about Mr P's story. The beginning of his life had been particularly difficult because although his mother had been able to take care of his practical needs, she was haunted by the ghost of her own psychotic mother and had a history of difficulties in maintaining relationships. She demanded care and attention from her son, and as the intellectually developed and cultured woman she was, she considered him to be like her and rewarded him from an early age for his learning achievements.

Moreover, his father was a man incapable of staying in a family dimension, a dimension perceived as a prison from which he escaped through long stays abroad and compulsive infidelity. It is possible that in this environment, watching became a way for Mr P to cling to the other and escape the constant danger of slipping into the various forms of emptiness enacted by his parents. He told me how his obsession with observing had initially had a creative and safeguarding impact on his life and had taken the form of an ability to use visual perception, free from symbolic thought, to draw and reproduce famous images and to memorise.[4] This latter ability had been rooted in his mother's expectations and had contributed to his academic success.

In the course of time, however, his obsession with watching took on different and more dangerous guises. At first, Mr P felt the urge to observe women at work and in the street; later, the obsession took the form of viewing internet pornography and compulsively searching for concrete erotic experiences.

Duck or rabbit

In gestalt theory, the image of a duck merging with a rabbit is an example of how visual perception uses a figural point (the rabbit's ears or the duck's beak) to orientate perception according to two different intentionalities, so that it is impossible to see the two images at the same time. Something similar happened in the analysis, where the two ways of considering the experiences recounted by Mr P oscillated in the analyst's mind between two paradigms. When Mr P shared his creative ability at work or his thoughts on a film or a book, the analyst could not help but notice the originality of his mind, the sensitivity with which he grasped aesthetic details and his ability to understand the other. But there were also times when he made the analyst aware of the predatory manner in which he regarded his partners, as soulless objects intended only for his pleasure. In those moments, the analyst felt a nagging sense of distance from him.

To reconcile this paradox, the analyst sometimes thought of Mr P as a perverse fetishist and that his other side was a bluff serving the sole purpose of covering up problematic behaviour. This viewpoint captured one aspect of his personality but did not exhaust its complexity.

Upon reflection, the analyst realised that she was adhering to the contradiction that Umberto Eco[5] had already formulated 50 years ago about modern and contemporary art. She was reliving something similar in the psychoanalytic situation.

One part of the public and critics sees in contemporary art only bluff, pure fetishism, while another part sees only creative and meaningful art.

Something similar has happened in psychoanalysis, where the field paradigm has reformulated many of the pivotal concepts that have formed the basis of therapy for over half a century. Despite the problematic reconciliation and integration of conceptual tools, in practice we live, with relative awareness, with two almost irreconcilable therapeutic paradigms.[6]

Using the *Diagnostic and Statistical Manual of Mental Disorders* categories, Mr P was a patient with a disordered personality and narcissistic and fetishistic traits. However, from a different perspective, Mr P was a severely traumatised patient whose symptoms could represent the analogue of an extreme cry for contact, at least bodily, with an "other" without the complication of feelings. To put it another way, he could sometimes consider the other as a subject, but there were times when he wished to regress to the phase in which the child uses the mother as an object capable of satisfying his omnipotent desire.

The analyst attempted to resolve this internal diatribe by adopting a philosophical stance; it was necessary to intervene in the categories through which thought takes shape: the scaffolding, definitions, narratives, mental experiments, images and implicit parables.

In other words she had to go deeply into the theoretical model she refers to: post Bionian field theory. She wondered why her mind was continually disturbed by thoughts stemming from a way of thinking aimed at establishing the kind of psychopathology she was facing. These thoughts were the defensive aspect through which the analyst tried to escape the fear of being overwhelmed or allowing herself to be used. On the way to bringing this oscillation into focus, the awareness of how something strange was happening to her compared to other analytic experiences was becoming increasingly evident. The first abnormal aspect she noticed was her lack of emotional involvement.

She thought this lack of feeling could somehow be related to the detachment Mr P referred to when he told her about his sexual encounters with prostitutes or the one-night stands that he did not wish to develop into relationships.

While understanding how the problematic relational situation was reproducing itself was of help, the idea of being, in the transference, the protagonist of a "pornographic" scene was a rather disturbing thought. And yet, not feeling meant that patient and analyst were staging, like the subjects of erotic performance, something that did not refer to anything else. On the contrary, they were in a relationship in which they were one and the same. Moreover, the style of speaking, the use of stark descriptions, was part of the radical spoliation that locked the relationship into a hyper-reality status.

L'Origine du monde and the origin of a transformation

Throughout the history of art, there have been many reproductions of nude figures, but none has caused more scandal than the oil on canvas painted by Gustave Courbet in 1866 entitled *L'Origine du monde*.[7] In the painting, there is a close-up depiction of the female genitalia, and this appears to be the most scandalous aspect. At the same time, the fact that the model is a faceless woman is only an insignificant detail.

Aside from the diatribe about what art is and how artistic representation differs from pornographic representation, what it is interesting to discuss in this context is the way in which reference to this painting in the analytic relationship facilitated a transition in the analyst's mind from hyper-realistic (pornographic) representation to artistic representation.

Mr P referred to Courbet's work, citing Jacques Lacan as the last owner of the painting. Based on this affiliation, he argued that the analyst seemed to censor his erotic practices when, like her famous colleague, she should have shared with him the pleasure of sexuality free from moral constraint. At least, this was how he interpreted Lacan's purchase of the work of art in question.

The impression the analyst got was not that he was enacting a seduction or distancing himself through irony but that he was asking her to look at things from his perspective and to see them as he did.

Mr P often emphasised how access to pornography and commitment-free sex was vital because it guaranteed two essential things: immediate fulfilment and the possibility of choosing how to feel fulfilled. In other words, everything was in his hands, and the other had to assume the same relational configuration as a mother with a very young child, giving him the illusion of creating the object[8] or, as Ogden proposed, of maintaining "the invisible oneness" (Ogden 1985, p. 250).[9]

The analyst trying to think instead offered him a continuous experience of painful dissonance.

Outside the session, she went back to look at the reproduction of Courbet's painting on the internet and came across news of how a Frenchman of letters had examined the correspondence between George Sand and Alexandre Dumas's son and noticed a transcription error[10] that allowed him to trace the identity of the model. Claude Schopp, author of the discovery, wrote a book about his research.[11]

What could it have meant to be with him, to share the same perspective? Was being faceless, i.e. without a head, thoughts and emotions, the way to be with him in the midst of catastrophe?

For years, psychoanalysis has investigated how early traumas can lead to structuring a profound "distortion of the essential processes fundamental to object relations".[12] Although the genital erotic theme is connected with an advanced stage of development, Mr P was enacting something that belonged to the early stages of emotional development[13].

The story of the painting and the ensuing dialogue in the session certainly brought patient and analyst closer to the relational drama that inhabited it, distancing the analyst from his defensive mechanisms which had been more prominent in the relational field in the early days.

The pain

A more violent explosion of pain erupted in the third year of treatment. Following a period of fierce quarrels between Mr P and his wife, which poisoned the atmosphere in the family, his eldest daughter attempted suicide. The potential loss of his daughter affected him more deeply than the estrangement from his wife while continuing to reside in the same house. As a result, his real-world erotic practices came to an abrupt halt, resuming online a few months later. It was during this time that he started telling the analyst about *Dipsea*, an erotic podcast he had recently discovered that soothed him more than the videos.

He told her that this service represented the future, as it already had 287 million users, and the company expected three billion subscribers within the next year.

Why did he feel the need to describe number of users in such detail and the supposed commercial fortunes of this unusual start-up? Why did he return to insignificant details that preceded and accompanied his evening connection to the podcast?

At first, I saw the fact that he had switched from video to audio as suggestive of a step toward a greater acceptance of therapy even though the reasons for it were not clear.

Did the idea that words mediated patient-analyst connection reassure her about not having to share the dissociated aspects of feeling that seemed to inhabit his obsession of watching porno videos?

Indeed, the ability of Mr P to listen more was accompanied by the feeling of being able to exist more as an analyst in the relationship, but she sensed and feared that this might only be a phase.

The fact that his narratives had become more and more filled with useless details made the analyst think, as Winnicott suggests, that Mr P had regressed to a phase of non-integration and that in analysis he was desperately trying to pick up the broken threads of his development.[14] His daughter's attempted suicide had intensely mobilised him on a relational level, so he, as the absent father he had been, now sought to provide opportunities for shared leisure time activities, especially involving music and concerts. These were special occasions for the developing relationship between them. Mr P seemed to provide his daughter with something he wanted for himself: a good rhythm that would allow a bond to be rebuilt.

Even with his daughter, however, the concert experience was imbued with a high level of excitement and transgression that Mr P described as belonging to "the animal in me".

The erotic podcasts seemed to have replaced the casual sexual encounters. The growing relationship between Mr P and his daughter and a climate of respite in the family seemed to be preconditions for developing a capacity to be in a relationship with the analyst.

After a few months, he resumed his meetings with prostitutes with whom something which neither he nor the analyst could have imagined manifested itself: impotence.

At first, it happened sporadically, allowing him to attribute it to external factors. As an example, he used to tell how certain work situations made him feel agitated, and anxiety could undoubtedly interfere with his body's ability to function.

He then began to complain increasingly about how using condoms disturbed him. He did not want to expose himself to the danger of contracting diseases, but he hated that "thing".

Listening to him, it struck the analyst that he hardly ever used the word "condom", opting instead for a word that left the semantic field open. This made it easier to wonder what it was that stood between patient and analyst that disturbed him so much and that was producing a painful loss of his sense of mastery and a distance between them in terms of being able to have a fulfilling experience.

The analyst explored many avenues to find a possible meaning with him: she suggested that their meetings, necessarily interspersed with days of not meeting, could make him feel the burden of being alone and managing something catastrophic without help. She made reference to how in his past, he had gone to great lengths to get close to his parents and how he had experienced a progressive sense of helplessness in achieving an emotionally satisfying relationship with them. Analyst and patient explored the hypothesis that what was happening to him could be a kind of message to help them understand better what stood in the way of fulfilment in his sexual relationships and the various facets of his life.

Mr P listened attentively but pointed out to the analyst that her thoughts were not only far from the truth but also ineffective. His feelings of helplessness became more frequent, and his anger towards her and psychoanalysis as being unable to help him, became more and more palpable. Mr P now shied away from sexual encounters, not because he no longer desired them, but because he was terrified of being confronted with an unacceptable experience of failure. What was becoming clear was that in the therapeutic relationship, the analyst also shared his sense of growing impotence, despair and sometimes non-contact.

Gaze and the animalistic side of experience

He adopted a dog abandoned by an acquaintance who had been forced to move and could not take the animal with him. The experience of loss and disorientation that he described when talking about the dog deeply echoed his own.

Moreover, during this period he began to reproduce Guernica and, in the session, he would tell the analyst how impressed he was by the horse's gaze and the mouth of the woman shattered by the death of the child lying in her arms. These bodily dimensions occupied a lot of time in the session, as if he were painting with words, moving towards and away from the figures so as to scrutinise their details. His descriptions evoked in the analyst the idea that he was exploring his primitive agonies through bodily brushstrokes on canvas. He described how Picasso had rendered the emotional experience not only through content but also through his painting style which was more or less distinct and pronounced in various parts of the painting. He also stressed repeatedly how fascinated he was by the painter's ability to compose an experience of both physical and psychic fragmentation within the space proposed by the painting.

He felt very lonely, and drawing absorbed him so much that he was able to set aside his troubles for a while.

The picture was at once an emotionally laden effort and a relief.

As he spoke about it, images of animals in other paintings came to the analyst's mind, particularly those by Caravaggio and Piero di Cosimo, two painters who embodied shadiness and emotional discontrol to almost legendary degrees. Both had painted an animal whose gaze captured something of the mute pain in the scene.

A dog occupies the right side of Piero di Cosimo's painting entitled *The Death of Procris*; with a sorrowful, questioning gaze, it sits staring at a dead girl lying on the lawn (see Figure 7.2).

The second image is the moist and vaguely disturbing eye of the donkey that appears almost suddenly in the background of Caravaggio's painting *Rest During the Flight into Egypt* (see Figure 7.3). While it is impossible to attribute undeclared intentions to the authors of these paintings, it seems as if both animals are bringing into the picture, through their gaze, that wordless pain that underlies experiences of uprooting, loss and distance; a pain that precedes consciousness and sometimes remains buried under anger, anti-social behaviour or acting out.

One evening when Mr P was working on reproducing the horse's gaze, which he said was so central to the Guernica painting and which he could not render as he would have liked, he looked up from the paper and met his dog's gaze. It was, he said, a breathtaking experience. He felt as if something other and alive was reaching him for the first time, a still indeterminate sensation that was nevertheless present even if mute, on the surface of the eye.

The dog's gaze took on a form far removed from any thought accessed through language, a way of looking at each other free from any fear or self-regard.

Mr P: The dog looked at me. It wanted nothing from me, it just looked at me and my looking at him seemed to be enough, without my reaching out to stroke or feed him.

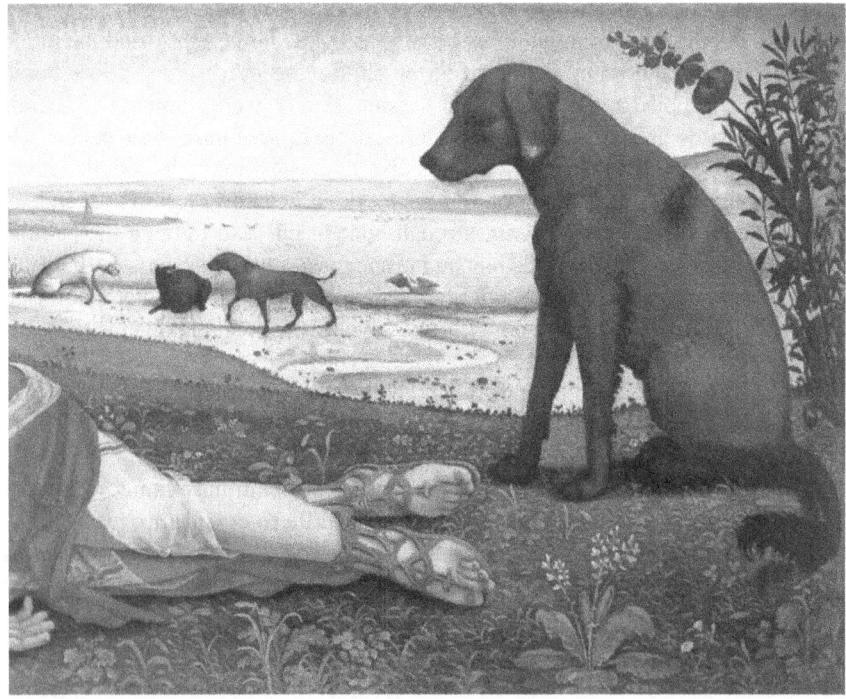

Figure 7.2 Piero Di Cosimo, *The Death of Procris* (detail).

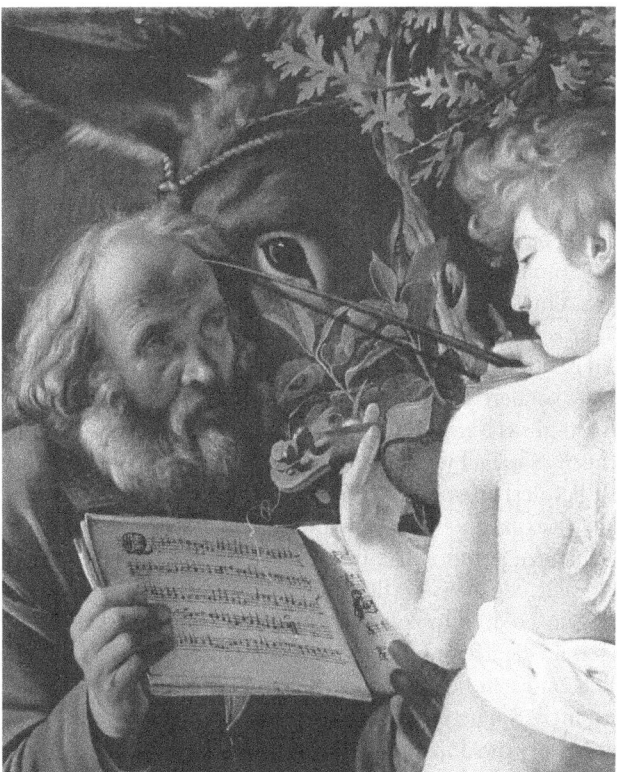

Figure 7.3 Caravaggio, *Rest on the Flight into Egypt* (detail).

Benjamin describes this kind of experience as an aura and writes that to be within the gaze is the implicit "expectation of being reciprocated by that to which it offers itself"[15]; the aura is what fills this expectation.

The dog's gaze overwhelmed him and did indeed create an aura and a breach in his defences. Their mutually raised gazes, which Benjamin described as creating "the unique apparition of a distance,"[16] enabled him to pause and enjoy this new kind of relationship rather than fleeing.

Perhaps he had reconnected with that developmental moment when an infant looks at the mother's face before thought could make the experience conscious and memorable.

In therapy, this reciprocity of gaze was reflected in a lessening of tension in the atmosphere which allowed analyst and patient to communicate with greater ease and sincerity.

The origin of the world and the end of analysis: a catastrophic transit

The therapeutic couple continued oscillating between moments of understanding and intimacy and moments of pain and disappointment until Mr P told the analyst he had to go abroad for work and be away for three months.

He did not agree to continue the therapy online but paid in advance for all the sessions he would miss. Halfway into that period, the analyst received a short message from Mr P telling that he was well and that he would resume meetings on his return.

During these three months, the analyst wondered what his relative disappearance and advance payment meant: at times, it seemed to be a prelude to the end of the analysis; at others, it seemed that it was premature to consider ending the analysis, and the advance payment was a way of keeping me tied to him. During that time, the analyst tried to maintain an attitude of confident expectation. He duly returned to the session, almost as if the thread of discourse had never been broken. He told that he had felt sincerely attracted to a colleague and had tried unsuccessfully to have a sexual relation with her.

The analyst wondered if whilst he was still abroad, Mr P had heard her brief SMS in reply to his as a resurfacing in analysis of the lack of maternal affection he had experienced. She had written: "Good. I'll see you as soon as you get back."

He added that despite spending the whole night with this woman, he had been unable to have sexual intercourse with her. But then, like a summer storm, the atmosphere changed abruptly. He raised the tone of his voice, quickened the pace of his words, and began to gesticulate in irrepressible rage. He told me that he was not going to be able to solve the problem through psychoanalysis, and that he would need medication or would try some other technique to solve his anxiety issue. He then said that he had found out that his problem of impotence affected about 25% of men. So, he concluded that what was happening to him could not be related to his history or subjectivity. It was a practical problem to which the analyst could not give an adequate answer.

The session ended in a stormy atmosphere in which the long-hypothesised anger had finally become tangible.

Patient and analyst were close but unable to have an emotionally fruitful experience of any kind.

At next meeting he appeared a little calmer and whilst attempting to go over the contents of the previous session, he told that, despite being aware that the analyst was now unable to help him, he was nonetheless grateful for the work done together and how it had helped him improve his social relationships and, above all, become a better father.

However, he also told, in a peremptory tone, that he would finish therapy at the beginning of the summer holidays, i.e. in two months' time. He had also contacted a private art school so that he could resume his old passion for drawing and have access to the technical equipment he needed to fully express his talent.

Over the next few days, the analyst felt dazed, unable to think and understand, pervaded only by a mixture of anxiety and helplessness. Then, somewhat ironically, she told herself that she was now included in that 25% of "men" with whom Mr P felt he belonged. The merit of this thought, however, lay in the fact that she was having the same feeling as her patient: not only the one that became evident in erotic encounters but also the ancient and profound feeling of being a child lost in an unbridgeable emotional distance in relationships with others.

She thought about the catastrophe of birth and how such a catastrophe can become ingrained in the psyche in the absence of another mind capable of helping the infant, through holding and reverie, to cope with the sensory and emotional hyper-stimulation of the external world, giving it back an experience of emotional containment and mediation of the enormous sensory stimulation. She remembered the painting *L'Origine du monde* we had talked about a year earlier.

It was intuitively clear how by establishing the end, Mr P had made the analyst the faceless model in the painting, the mother without a mind, the unloving and unloved wife.

Above all, it seemed possible that Mr P's erasure of the analyst restituted his sense of hold on the other and the world that had allowed him to survive through looking.

The sense of sight had been the medium through which he had avoided psychic death and had allowed him to discover his ability to create the absent object. As he struggled with a situation of despairing helplessness, he tried to retrace the path that had, at least in part, saved him from catastrophe. Once again, he felt he had to do everything himself: get rid of the analyst and enrol in an art school.

In a session during which the analyst felt like crying the way Mr P had done at their first meeting, a feeling she was now also trying to hold back by blowing her nose and piling up tissues at the edge of the chair, she tried to share these thoughts with him.

She told him that by eliminating her "blah blah", perhaps he could return to that condition where words do not exist except as rhythm and sound and where seeing had been an essential and saving experience for him. Moreover, eliminating her could mean emancipating himself from that mother who demanded him to be through academic performances and against whom he had rebelled through the body.

Now that his body had failed him, he was once again assailed by feelings of despair, and his distancing himself from words and what the analyst had partly reproduced seemed to offer him a means of salvation.

In particular, not seeing the analyst anymore would allow his gaze to find new footholds.

There was a long painful silence. When Mr P spoke, he said that he had not considered analyst's words as "blah blah" and was sorry for giving her the impression that he did not appreciate the road they had travelled together. In the next session, he said that things had got out of hand when he told he was thinking about ending his analysis and realised only now how he had become exaggeratedly furious. The thought of ending the analysis had occurred to him a few months earlier, but he had kept it jealously to himself, sharing it with very few friends. As was the case with Courbet's painting, the various owners who had bought it over time had chosen to keep it hidden and only shared it with their closest friends.

In the painting, it was not the hyper-realism of the representation that was so difficult to share but the catastrophe of a hyper-real representation of a living object as opposed to a subject.[17]

Moreover, in its title the painting alludes to birth and the complicated dependency everyone experiences with their mother.

In the remaining weeks of therapeutic time, the analyst decided to stay close to him and convey, as best she could, the idea that the end of his analysis was probably the transit through which he was about to reach another condition of life within himself.

She told him that making her disappear was perhaps the way he would begin to see her from another point of view and how this could be the beginning of a further change.

Although the analyst felt pain, she was also aware that as happens during the birth process, from that moment on, analyst and patient would be separate and committed to inventing a relationship capable of replacing the previous one, and she hoped that for Mr P it would be different from the one previously practised through his obsession with pornography. In short, the "loving" connection they had shared in the analytical relationship would guarantee an imperfect separation, never completely radical, perhaps repairing the experience he had had during his childhood.

Mr P had missed out on this experience, so the fracturing of the early mother-infant symbiotic bond became a void in which only the sight seemed to offer him a chance to retrace something of the old bond. So, through images that remained implicit in the analyst's mind, she tried to share with him the potential leap he was about to take. The painful and one-sided surprise of his decision to keep her in the dark was an epilogue in which aspects of birth and the old ways he had treated all his partners were mixed.

What made the analyst inclined to give credence to the first hypothesis was that in the sessions following the announcement of his decision to terminate when they spoke so intimately about their feelings, the atmosphere became very different and more mutually caring.

In the last sessions, the analyst felt sure he was heartened not to feel blamed and to be experiencing, to a certain extent, in the analytical relationship what he had probably only partly experienced in the relationship with his mother: recognition as a subject in his own right. Mr P had re-experienced the merging of goodness seen and goodness perceived; he arrived with a cake he had made by himself and invited the analyst to celebrate, in their respective homes, the end of the therapeutic relationship or as he put it, the beginning of his new life: his re-birthing. As he handed the analyst the cake on the doorstep, they looked each other in the eye, just as had happened for the first time with his dog.

Becoming "O"

"In psychoanalytic practice, 'looking at' is inseparable from experiencing of 'turbulence'."[18] With this sentence, Bion relates the connecting experience in the distance (looking at) to the experience of subjectivation. During early development, the achievement of an awareness of being intimately related yet separate from the mother entails a complex process that is laden with uncertainty. It requires the baby to experience a sufficiently solid relationship in which the mother can offer herself as a container for his anxieties and actively help him transform them.

During psychoanalysis, this process recurs and is made more distressing by the deployment of defences that have protected the core self from disintegration. In Mr P's many accounts of his erotic life, the act of looking was disengaged from emotional engagement and often only functional to achieve a solitary orgasm. He sometimes and ironically referred to the blindness myth used to dissuade people from masturbating. It was an attempt to control sexuality and, to this day, only a belief of the past. However, transposed to the analytic relationship, masturbation can be understood as a practice in which the analyst or the patient keep themselves at a safe distance from an experience of deep mental coupling, a practice that can also provide particular intellectual pleasure, e.g. in establishing connections, developing hypotheses and reconstructing personal history. However, before working with Mr P, the analyst had never reflected on the measure of emotional truth in this old wives' tale that echoes the ontological shift currently taking place within psychoanalysis.[19] It means that the most critical transformation to be pursued is the transformation in O, that is, a fundamental commitment to the principle of being and becoming in the experience rather than an epistemological exploration.

Therefore, transformation in O is a new experience that can only "become" at a non-differentiated level in the transference, at a deep level of mental coupling. This proposition is not only functional to theoretical speculation but also the level necessary to address the challenge of those early traumatic residues that did not have access to signification never having gone beyond bodily experience. There remain sensations buried in the body, in the acts, in the self-harming compulsion that barely find the mnemonic and meaning link that can reconnect them to experience.

Being a psychoanalyst with Mr P, therefore, entailed for some time no longer being a psychoanalyst, experiencing the darkness of exclusion from sharing, accepting to be exposed to a pornographic relationship, that is, one in which intimacy is a-relational.

For a long time, the way Mr P used analysis was reminiscent of Courbet's faceless model, forcing an ontologically relational therapeutic experience towards the repetition of emptiness and blindness, in which he could, for the most part, share the defensive setup that had protected him from psychic catastrophe. Blindness, like other catastrophic transits, is one of those experiences that are "indescribable"[20] as "being" something is different from "understanding it".[21] What was barely describable was the return to sharing a level where the patient used the analyst as an object until he could find the mirror of himself in the other's gaze.

In this analysis, it was possible to cross the threshold that connects and separates us as human beings from the animal kingdom. The reference to animality was a theme to which Mr P had referred at the beginning of the analysis to describe the instinctual drive that drove him towards erotic intercourse and later to recount the new experience he was having with his dog.

He discovered how the dog reciprocated his affective impulses and never sought revenge for his neglect. On the contrary, his dog was faithful to him, he said, and then added with irony, "not like me." Yet it was through this loyalty and the experience of persistence of the object that analysis offered him, Mr P discovered his humanity. Mr P regarded the women with whom he tried to have sexual relations with the ambivalence and estrangement through which humans sometimes distance themselves from the animal kingdom: women, like animals, had a body but were not a body. In this split is the violence of a way of thinking in which human beings, distinguished by their capacity for language and self-consciousness, feel unique and superior. In Mr P's case, all the violence of being unable to discover himself depended on the other. This position guaranteed Mr P the same feeling of superiority and omnipotence, but at a deeper level, this predatory mode revealed envy and anger about not being able to experience his corporeity and sexuality without anguish.

However, towards the end of the analysis, the first exchange of glances between him and his dog allowed him to cross that subtle threshold; he experienced the aura that connects and separates humans and animals, and this aura opened a crack in his way of protecting himself from the other.

Mr P initially reassured himself by maintaining a distance up until the moment we faced what was happening.

We explored his anguish through words and experienced being together. O became the vertex from which to look at what we were experiencing.

Bion writes, "The analyst cannot be identified with this vertex; he must be this vertex."[22] The erasure of the analyst achieved this perspective.

Notes

1 Bancalari 2015.
2 Fornari 1982.
3 Winnicott describe this developmental step in "The use of an object and relating through identifications", 1969, p. 355–364.
4 In a famous manual entitled *Drawing with the Right Brain*, Betty Edwards (1981) proposes a method and a series of strategies to "trick" the left hemisphere, which tends to be dominant, and allow the right hemisphere to "direct operations". This makes it possible to obtain results that are very faithful to what is observed.
5 Eco (1964) argued that the Manichean dichotomy between classic and modern art was triggered by the conflict between high and mass culture to which the two types of art were destined. Starting in those years, however, the paradigm seems to have been reversed. Here paradigm is used in a sense proposed in the scientific world by Tomas S. Kuhn (1962). However, in psychoanalysis, as in art, scientific paradigms are not as impermeable as in science, and different paradigms can long coexist because the community involved is much broader and less compact than the scientific one. Therefore, speaking of emerging and/or dominant paradigms in a given historical context would be correct.
6 Here, paradigm is used in the sense proposed in the scientific world by Thomas S. Kuhn (1962). However, in psychoanalysis, as in art, scientific paradigms are not as impermeable as in science, and different paradigms can coexist because the community involved is much broader and less compact than the scientific one. Therefore, speaking of emerging and/or dominant paradigms in a given historical context would be correct.
7 Due to its explicit non-idealised content, the painting passed through the hands of several collectors and was exhibited only in private contexts until 1995. It was then acquired by the French State and exhibited at the Musée d'Orsay. Publicly sharing the image on the internet, however, continues to generate reactions of censorship and denunciation (see the recent Facebook case of persecution of a French teacher).

8 Winnicott 2017a.
9 Ogden 1985, p. 250.
10 "One cannot paint Mademoiselle Queniault's interview with one's most delicate and musical brush". The word *interieur* was mistranslated as *anterview* instead of *intimate parts*.
11 Schopp (2018) discovered that the model in question was Mademoiselle Constance Queniault, a dancer at the Paris Opera. She agreed to pose for her lover, Khalil Bay, a wealthy Parisian of Turkish origin.
12 Winnicott 2017c, 1963, p. 105.
13 Glover 2009.
14 Winnicott 1945.
15 Benjamin 1997, p. 147.
16 Benjamin 1999, pp. 514–515, 526–527.
17 Benjamin 2004. In this Book the author explore the Third in early development through the movement between recognition and breakdown.
18 Bion 1975, p. 107.
19 Eshel 2017, 2019; Ogden 2019; Katz 2016.
20 Bion 2013, p. 85.
21 Bion 1991, pp. 182–183.
22 Bion 1970, pp. 40–41.

Chapter 8

Seeking comfort in an uncomfortable chair

I will use the word "comfort", that is an unusual word in the psychoanalytical dictionary, to explore the intersection between two tools of therapeutic technique and their utility in sustaining transformation: the couch and the chair. These two tools, for a long time, have contributed to the distinction between psychoanalysis and psychotherapy: exploring comfort is a way to analyse the distinction between these two ways of taking care of the patients, and to ask ourselves whether theoretical concepts used to distinguish them are still useful.

The "down side" of the uncomfort mentioned in the title refers to, in a global way, the difficulty of controlling emotional turbulence for both the analyst and the patient whatever the setting in which they meet is.

Bruno Munari, a designer in 1944, was the first in his field to ask himself what kind of relation there may be between originality and comfort in the design of a new piece of furniture and the aim to design beautiful but comfortable objects. With his signature humour, he wrote:

> A man goes back home after having worked all day, and finds an uncomfortable chair.[1]

From this sentence, and in particular from a sequence of pictures in which we can see Munari seeking comfort in an uncomfortable chair, comes the need to explore how the tools of the setting allow the patients to have a comforting experience, aiming to transform the psychic fatigue that urges them to ask for help. In order to do this we will use the intuition that spawns from experience to extract the meaning of the experience itself, as in the phenomenological method.

We therefore use the concept of comfort in relation with the setting, which is the way in which we can welcome the patient through analytical experience, with the goal of exploring the line between psychotherapy and psychoanalysis from a relational point of view, and in particular understanding how comfort and transformation can depend on each other.

The word comfort won't be used to describe something that belongs to the analyst or the patient, the conscious or the unconscious, the healthy or the unhealthy, but we use this word as a probe to analyse the balancing point, which Bion refers to as *caesura*.[2]

DOI: 10.4324/9781003388838-9

The distinction between psychotherapy and psychoanalysis that had resulted in different tools in each of these experiences had been useful in the past, but now we must start thinking about it through new theoretical concepts.[3]

In the past psychotherapy was a low-frequency therapy, performed face to face, where the analyst's sentences were intended to sustain the Ego of the patient. Analytical experience was a therapy with a high session frequency, where the patient would be on the couch, and the analyst's interpretations are more metaphorical and more directed to explore the unconscious.[4]

The use of the couch, which involves an experience of sensory deprivation, which is mostly uncommon in everyday life, was indicated as suitable for patients with a personality structure that wasn't too fragile and as an essential tool to enable the "analytic couple".[5]

The use of the couch and the high frequency of sessions have became for many analysts two inseparable aspects in the praxis. Having three or four sessions a week may be quite uncommon, yet it is surely more useful, but it may seem overwhelming for many people.

We must admit some low number session therapies may still deliver important transformation, on the other hand, in some cases standard analysis is either interrupted or for whatever reason doesn't result in any major improvement.[6]

We can't consider frequency as one of the most important transformation-inducing factors.[7]

Many personal factors, for example the clash between different personalities, or the availability of thinking tools, can condition the outcome of therapy.

In this complexity, the idea of putting together the concept of comfort with that of the setting, aims to explore the caesura between psychotherapy and psychoanalysis starting from an everyday life point of view.

Comfort yesterday and today

Apart from the patients who knew analytic experience indirectly and students of psychotherapy schools, people who ask to be helped rarely consider the outcome of going through a high-frequency therapy on the couch. Common experience tells us that at the onset of serious symptoms, the patient's desire is to begin therapy with one or two weekly sessions. Being an analyst who has personally been through analytical experience and witnessed the rewards of an intensive mental contact, the desire is to offer the patient a similar experience. This desire can be mitigated, ruled by considerations of opportunity, availability, psycho diagnostic assessments, and sometimes deviated from unconscious reluctance but, as a matter of fact desire does exist. Balancing these two points of view has always been far from easy. This distinction and the condensation of the difference in precise elements have emerged throughout the history of psychoanalytic movement. Its roots can be found in Freud's need to release the treatment process from the subjective qualities of the analyst in order to direct the treatment closer to the scientific paradigm.

The edge on which the question has arisen, that is the role of subjectivity, went dissolving progressively because accredited theories and authors have made the edge itself obsolete: the theory of Bion and post Bion, the infant research and psychoanalysis relational research.

However, in a recent conference, a leading exponent of the theory of post Bion restated, through a metaphor of love, the old judgment value between the two methods: psychoanalysis would embody the fullness of love, whereas psychotherapy is closer to the preliminary engagement of a love relationship. Sometimes, in the group situations, the unconscious adherence to ideas for the shape in which they occur resurface resembling "basic assumptions" forgetting Anna Freud words highlighting the relation between theory and technique in the analyst's outlook:

> [Variations of the technique] are occasioned, not by a change in the type of disorder treated, but by a change in the analyst's outlook and theoretical evaluation of familiar phenomena. The intimate interrelation between theory and practice in psychoanalysis is responsible for the fact that every development in theory results inevitably in a change of technique.
>
> (A. Freud 1954, p. 608)

The tools such as those that promote the transformation in a dream and allow the observation of the relationship in its micro textual and bodily components, have a use value in their transformative effectiveness and not in the frequency with which they have the opportunity to use them.[8]

Exploring comfort

Using the concept of comfort to choose a setting which is good enough for both the patient and the analyst and in particular considering the therapeutic value of this choice, we need to describe, from a psychic and therapeutic point of view, what comfort is. So as a starting point we can use body experience as it is the most intuitive.

We can say that feeling comfortable in a chair means leaning back, staying on a pillow which is neither too hard nor too soft and having the possibility to change position.

Furthermore, the body experience of comfort, as suggested by Munari, moves away from aesthetic concepts and from the accession to the needs of social or intellectual belonging, so to then return close to the simpler needs of daily life, to the desires of that particular moment in life.

A further consideration is that comfort is not a quality that is exclusive to the object but originates from the encounter that takes into account the needs at that time.

If you have back pain, a soft and wrapping chair, which is normally a comfortable chair, becomes at that time a means of intensifying the pain itself.

From a physical point of view the idea of comfort is simple and intuitive yet complex and multifaceted.

In order to feel comfortable in the analytic experience, the patient needs a good emotional restraint, a contact that allows the patient to explore the conscious and unconscious workings of the mind in a relationship that meets the needs of that moment in life.

These complex functions are rooted in the experience of the body which finds its origins in the rhythm and space of the meetings, has communicated through a preverbal channel and has its roots in procedural unconsciousness.

Finally, from the physical experience, that is the experience of a body moving to find an optimal adaptation between itself and the object, comes the consideration that comfort is not a state but a tendency towards a condition that is both stable for the time being, yet unstable in time.

In conclusion moving the point of view from the instrument to its use in the analytical couple, the concept of comfort is useful to describe the experience of the complex relationship which supports the analytical experience.

To describe more precisely what constitutes the concept of psychic comfort and how it can be used, I describe how this idea blends with some theoretical concepts.

Comfort and body-mind relationship

In his last work *Memory of Future*, Bion writes:

> I may be in error to discriminating between "mental" phenomena and "physical" facts. Such an "idea" is perhaps a flaw in the mental apparatus. As a human I have a prejudice in favour of regarding my thoughts as "superior" to the apparently random movements of infinitely minute particles of matters?
>
> (1979, p. 265)

This reference helps us understand how the body, along with emotions, are key elements in Bion's theory. The experience of the body participates actively and continuously to the genesis of thought, and it's the body itself that provides the raw material destined to be transformed into elements of psychoanalysis.

The body in the session is not in the field of thought but neither in the concrete. It often hosts a pre-mental dimension that is about to produce thought.

The body is the element from which a new thought can spawn, a thought that has yet to arise.

We must therefore consider that the body image is not intended as the element capable of generating communication elements subordinated to symbolic thought and speech.[9]

The observations arising from neuroscience strengthen the role and the importance of sensory perception and movement as important elements in the construction of the unconscious system. The sensory patterns are in fact an expression of an integrated experience of which we are not aware, that we use as a basis in the search for emotional consonance.[10]

In this context the observation of Frances Tustin on how autistic children find it difficult to pass from feeling to its relational *unconscious* use, looks very acute and useful for our discourse:

"To help you to understand it, try a little experiment" – writes – "Forget your chair. Instead, feel your seat pressing against the seat of the chair. It will make a shape. If you wriggle, the shape will change. Those "shapes" will be entirely personal to you".[11]

(Tustin 1986, p. 125)

Although impossible to deliver in words, feelings are commonly used unconsciously to fit the body, posture and tone, seeking personal comfort and conditioned by emotions of pleasure and by the posture of other's bodies. The countless investigations around the observation of a premature baby-mother, then transposed in the therapeutic relationship with an adult, clearly showed how our bodies will play a role of intense relationship in a nonverbal way, a kind of dance relational albeit remote. This emotional, procedural and unconscious operating model, learned in the primary relationship, becomes a kind of style to which we relate to others, but it is also able to evolve throughout life and to build moments of contact also implicitly shared with subjects with different relational patterns.[12]

Returning to the initial quote which connects "physical" and "psychological" is interesting that he not only establishes a relationship between the two parameters but keeps them in power, in the relationship of oscillation which is one of the most original and creative elements of Bion's theory and its developments.

Mind: Hullo! Where have you sprung from?
Body: What – you again? I am Body; you can call me Soma if you like. Who are you?
Mind: Call me Psyche – Psyche-Soma.
Body: Soma-Psyche
Mind: We must be related
Body: Never – not if I can help it.
Mind: Oh, come. Not as bad as that, is it?

(Bion 1979, p. 433)

Considering the relationship body-mind from this point of view, an idea is not only a flaw in complexity of the "matter" but something in the flowing of the matter. So Bion's hypothesis that beta elements, the raw feelings and emotions in a primitive state, are transformed into alpha elements, the basis of thought through dream work, has been expanded. The assumption is that this transformation can not only have a one-way sense but alpha and beta stay in never-ending oscillation between each other. This sort of mathematical equation can be seen as a theoretical synthesis of the complex interaction of mind and body.[13] Like the unconscious, through the permeability of the contact barrier, deconstructs and makes creative consciousness, so tone and movement posture allow the procedural unconscious to establish a contact with the body of the other in an adaptive relation that swings endlessly.

Returning to the chair and its comfort, we can say that the chair that the analyst offers contains the complex experience of how it greets the patient. The chair unconsciously communicates, through form, something about the analyst and his perception of the patient's unconscious patterns.

The concept of comfort or rather its pursuit, captures this need for subsequent adjustments over time within a relationship between the analyst and the patient.

As in everyday life, a feeling of comfort is a starting point to do something else, so the comfort and psychic relationship are the basis for affective consonance, the production of images, dreams and thoughts from which stories and narration spawn and take form.

Comfort and binocular vision

Through the term *binocular vision*, Bion intended to describe an aspect of the psychoanalytic method, starting from a physical experience.

Each eye sees the object from a distinct perspective and has the need to accommodate, that is, to find the right distance between itself and the object through the modification of the curvature of the anterior surface of the lens and the adjustment of the light through the ciliary muscle that determines the diameter of the pupil. An "optimal distance" between the two vertices of view is also needed, so they can converge towards the same picture, giving the subject a perception of depth.

In the beginning Bion[14] described binocular vision as a necessary point of view to take care of psychotic patients. They present material that cannot be interpreted only as effects of psychological development divorced from physical development. There are parts of psychotic personality (proto-mental system) in which mental and physical states are undifferentiated.

Evolving his ideas, Bion used the concept of binocular vision to describe the need to proceed in the analytic work, keeping in mind the relationship between the conscious and the unconscious. This opportunity is ensured by the smooth functioning of an intra-subjective function he called contact barrier. Focus depends on whether the alpha elements, the result of the work of transformation of feelings and raw emotions, guarantee the right distance and proximity between these two ways of thinking.[15]

Through the same *binocular vision* term, Bion described the usefulness to the group analyst to maintain the view of a double focus: the way each component's interior group works, and the one that is generated between players in the same group.[16]

Binocular vision may finally be a descriptor of the analytic bi-personal situation in which the analyst and the patient both have a personal perspective from which to try to understand the experience in which they are involved.

What I want to emphasise (and which intersects with the idea of comfort) is the fact that only when analyst and patient reach an optimal "distance/proximity" between conscious and unconscious functioning between themselves and their inner group and in their relationship, is there the possibility of a focused and deeper vision.

The interpretation, the instrument considered for characterising psychoanalysis, has been for a long time the main tool to get the optimal emotional proximity. It has undergone a profound transformation going from a mainly revealing use of an unconscious truth foreseen by the analyst to a formulation of a hypothesis of provisional sense and subject to the possibility of being accepted and used by the patient. Psychoanalysis has become less interpretative and more narrative, and the expansion of "thinkability" is the real goal of the therapy.

In this change, the analyst takes care of the comfort of the patient avoiding the "violence" of unipersonal interpretation.

The same evolutionary process can be envisioned for the use of the couch or chair and the frequency of sessions. They may be the subject of a binocular vision that does not mean a compromised vision but a vision that is confronted with the concept of the right distance/proximity to focus on those conscious and unconscious phenomena that arise in the analytic relationship.

These concrete aspects of the setting combine to determine the ease and quality of a shared vision.

Their preference of both subjects of the analysis depends on the ability of each to adapt to the curvature of their visual. The ability to change position in the chair is described as one of the aspects that determine the experience of comfort. From a psychic point of view, it could mean to abandon psycho-diagnosis, which is a tool in a one-person vision, and propose the use of the couch and frequency without exercising constraints. We can consider these instrument settings as functions of the intersubjective contact barrier. By intersubjective contact barrier I mean the conscious and unconscious experience that is created, moment by moment, in the relationship and in its ongoing mutual adaptations.

The desire of each of the two subjects and patients in particular on the possibility to either see or not see each other during the session and the frequency of the meetings should be viewed as emerging conscious and unconscious elements to observe, accept and dream about together.

Comfort and intersection with O-K

The concept of "O" in Bion's theory has different meanings: the thing itself, similar to Kant's unknowable reality *noumen*, the emotional unison in the relationship, the aspect that transcends "Human" therefore something that only those who are open to mystical knowledge can approach.

What margin of the concept of comfort may intercept O?

In a way we can assume that the word *comfort* is a description of something about the patient's emotional experience of unison with himself and those with the analyst during the analytic session.

The experience of unison ("at-one-ment") is an important source of experience and personality growth. Bion suggested that the experience of unison can swing between moments of profound harmonic consciousness (K) and sensory and emotional moments of harmony in which you approach and grasp fragments of unknowable reality.

I hypothesise that the idea of being comfortable intersects the concept of harmony in K or O in the most dynamic instance, where K is transformed into O and O into K.

In dynamic movement described by the double arrow, the feeling of comfort tends to break more or less extensively to give way to the discovery of a new comfort asset. The comfort turns into discomfort, emotional unison, mental and physical harmony is achieved that later breaks to then allow O to get back in swing with K. We can therefore imagine there are moments of comfort that is an experience that relates to the physical and emotional knowledge and experience in K or in O, but both are quite suddenly inhabited by an experience of discomfort that favours the disintegration, so then to reorganise itself in another place in the field.

Different points of view

I will explain three different clinical situations in which comfort is viewed from different points of view.

What joins them is the path that brings the two subjects to seek comfort within the analysis as an element capable of promoting transformation in the mind.

From the patient's perspective

When Beckett was 27 years old he was a fairly unknown and humanly depressed writer. In an effort to quarantine a state that seems to lead "to the depths of madness", he comes into contact with Dr. Wilfred R. Bion at the Tavistock Clinic. He stayed on therapy with Bion for about two years. During this period he started writing his first novel, *Murphy* and completed it a year after he ended the relationship with Bion.

Regarding the therapy, we know something by a fragment of an interview released in 1989 by Beckett himself and reported in James Knowlson's biography:

> I used to lie down on the couch and try to go back in my past. I think it probably did help. I think it helped me perhaps to control the panic. I certainly came up with some extraordinary memories of being in the womb. Intrauterine memories. I remember feeling trapped, of being imprisoned and unable to escape, of crying to be let out, no one could hear, no one was listening. I remember being in pain but being unable to do anything about it.
>
> (Knowlson 1996, p. 171)

Beckett, referring to the womb of the mother, alludes to the desire to rebirth but also the profound sense of entrapment that characterised the relationship with his mother. This was one of the most painful and difficult aspects of his therapy. The voltage generated by the thrust of Bion to facilitate the detachment and Beckett's inability to actually do so, was the likely cause of the rupture of their therapeutic relationship.

We can therefore assume that what Beckett refers to his mother is the same feeling he got from Bion.

During the therapy sessions, Bion himself suggested Beckett should write in order to release pain and inner struggle. So, during his therapy, Beckett starts writing his first novel, *Murphy*, whose protagonist holds many clear references to the writer's actual life and problems:

> He sat naked in his rocking-chair of undressed teak, guaranteed not to crack, warp, shrink, corrode, or creak at night. It was his own, it never left him. . . . Seven scarves held him in position. . . . Only the most local movements were possible. Sweat poured off him, tightened the thongs his entire body. The breath was not was perceptible. The eyes, cold and unwavering as gull's, started up at an iridescence splashed over the cornice moulding, shrinking and fading.
>
> (Beckett 1938, p. 3)

What is interesting and emerges clearly in the novel is how the fact of being caged and divided is not only in the relationship with the mother but also in the one with Bion.

The choice of a rocking chair highlights the desire of being lulled, of a rhythm of ancestral peace, the need for a swing that turns creeks, nightmares and defects of his psychological structure.

The desire to be free contrasts with Murphy's description of binding himself to the chair with seven bands. There is an image of condensed need of containment (bands), of an attempt of self-containment that mingles with self-imprisonment.

Later in the novel Beckett captures the widening chasm that lives within himself, and to express it more clearly as it steps into a painful separation of body and mind:

> Thus Murphy felt himself split in two, a body and a mind. They had intercourse apparently, otherwise he could not have known that they had anything in common. But he felt his mind to be bodytight and did not understand trough what channel the intercourse was effected nor how the two experience came to overlap. He was satisfied neither followed from the other.
>
> (Beckett 1938, p. 68)

More than in therapy Beckett seems to have benefited from the writing as a kind of self-analysis seeking to transpose into the novel the pace, style and shape of the analytical process.[17]

Conversely the influence of Beckett penetrated to some extent in the work of Bion that approached literature to the extent of making, at the end of his life, the form to which entrusts his personal story and the accumulated analytical experience.

In the analysis between Bion and Beckett, we can capture Beckett's difficulty in feeling comfortable in the relationship with Bion and how only later they found in the aesthetic form of literature a meeting place capable of containing the anguish and transforming it through shared narrative at a distance in time and space.

Obviously contextualising the relationship in a time when many analytical instruments had not yet been developed, we do not intend to assume a position of judgment but only to show how this masterly literary example of gathering the essence of the experience of comfort and discomfort as a complex experience of psychophysical type, finds a relatively simple expression of talking about daily experience.

From the analyst perspective

In the first session Silvano tells how his life was marked by tragedy at the end of adolescence: he used his parents' car to go to school on a freezing winter day. He lost control of the car and went on the other side of the street killing another person.

Many years passed before emerging from this tragedy and now life rages again with him, denying the joy of a child. Perhaps for this failure the relationship with his wife is going through a crisis.

By binding to this he extracts the phone and shows me a picture of him, a bit blurry, which acts as a screen saver. He explains that the night before he had a serious argument with his wife because he had replaced the picture of himself and his wife together with the one that just pictured himself. He explains that the photo in question, which shows him out of focus, while he is moving to the camera, reflects his feeling better than the picture where he was posing with his wife.

Only for a brief moment I thought that death and the desire for a new life were among us, and I wondered what this desire to eliminate the stereotyped couple was, but it's a fleeting intuition that I do not know how to use.

At the end of the intake sessions, we discussed the formal aspects of our analytic contract. He desires to come twice a week, but he cannot pay the amount that I am charging. He tells me the most he can afford is six meetings a month. He is very aggressive, and he anticipates that he doesn't want to come once a week because he knows that it would be useless. He wants me to change my honorary. The analytic therapy is suddenly exposed to the possibility of falling in the bud and the deathly crash is now in the room. As with his wife, I feel removed from the screen and my chair is suddenly covered with sharp shards of glass on which I feel very uncomfortable.

I tell him that I do not agree to change the conditions of the contract but, until the summer, namely for four months, he will not pay the two session missing in his budget.

A moment later, I say to myself that the solution is very bad; I would have been overwhelmed by his sudden change of tone, from how I felt surprised and angry, but at this point I cannot accept myself moving like him in the photo.

When I use in my mind the word *overwhelmed*, my mind goes back to the accident, as his survival coincided with the death of the other, as in him there is a sincere desire for a new life but, for that to happen, we must learn to be an analytic couple.

The next session he spontaneously asked me to use the couch on which he says he will feel "more comfortable". In the coming months I have to find a new comfort in my chair, a condition passing through the processing of violent, raw emotions, sometimes sharp as splinters. I am conscious, although it's hard to accept it, that the initial compromise played a role, not only in the sense of avoiding the crash.

The uncomfort of my chair and his choice of the couch as a comfortable element of the setting, the cut of my honorary as an expression of an excessive emotional cost, the oscillation between the meeting and his need to kill me have played an important role in the therapy. Many times when we have talked again, the allusion to comfort and uncomfort has returned as an experience that encompasses physical and mental factors.

A binocular vision

Sara, back from a short break we had agreed upon following the birth of her child, told me that she needed to bring her baby to one of our three weekly sessions. I assumed that my patient had a number of reasons to have her child in the session: her partial difficulty dealing with separation and something regarding the relation with me that we will discover together in the following sessions.

When I agreed with her request, I did not imagine that it was not concerning only that one session. To my surprise, the following week she came again with her baby and this new arrangement went on for a few months.

Whilst the first time, the child sat confortly in his baby's chair, making his presence felt with some wails, his presence gradually became more obvious.

I invited the young mother to change the setting and to use the armchair to hold the child in her arms in a more comfortable way. She refused my offer because switching position was too difficult for her.

So we started to speak together about the body, its position, the difficulty of changing and the problem of feeling comfort and discomfort in the chair or on the couch.

The patient started saying that she felt as if her child distracted us so much that she experienced the session as a waste of time and money.

It was hard for both of us to restructure our space, planned for two, and to make it flexible so as to adjust it to an ever-changing situation.

However, to grasp the usual setting was probably a way to prevent ourselves from evolving thought to something new.

I kept on wondering why we both – probably for different reasons – wanted the baby between us and if the baby can be thought of as something new birthing in the analytical relationship.

So, we continued to use the old setting – she on the couch and I in the chair behind her – for all the sessions. The second session of the week started with the patient lying on the couch, then she would stand up to take the crying child on her lap, and sometimes the most practical solution was to breastfeed him.

I observed the mother and her child in a position that looked very uncomfortable, and I would end up feeling just as uncomfortable in an armchair all for myself.

The traditional setting that the patient felt as something she just could not give up was now a limitation in talking and dreaming. The child was in the same time something new and a form of constraint, and we had to discover it as a psychoanalytical fact.

The issue of the double register that more evidently regarded the setting of the sessions at some point felt to me as also concerning the kind of dialogue in the three-person sessions. At times both the mother and I were able to maintain dialogue by putting the child aside, without really excluding him. At other times the presence of the child attracted our attention, and we were both reaching out to him, making hypotheses about the kind of need he expressed non-verbally. When this happened, we both experienced a diversion from the discourse unfolding between the two of us.

It seemed to me that the continuity ensured by the patient with her child while she was talking with me was also a particularly valuable experience for her, as she had gone through dramatic and repeated affective disruptures during her life. The child, being a person in his own right and not only a part of the infantile self, exerted a creative twist on this issue.

The experience of again finding some continuity in discontinuity, that at first was a challenge in alternating different settings, also appeared in the session, and the capacity to manage and integrate verbally and non-verbally what happened implied an effort in a new direction. What seemed to slowly emerge was that in the three-person sessions we began to experience some overlapping freedom and emphasis on the value of nonverbal communications and images that were different from the classic sessions.

When the patient after some months was able to stand up from the armchair and the three of us could sit on the mat together, she said that she felt pleasantly well. This new feeling was not stemming from something I did or said, but from her capacity to play with her infantile self within and without (Bloom 2000). She recalled a dream from the beginning of her analysis where *she and I were eating a sandwich together, sitting on the mat*. A dream that at that time, in the midst of intense emotional storminess, had seemed a dreamlike relational heaven.

Since that session the patient stopped bringing her child to the sessions informing me she had found someone who would take care of the infant during her sessions.

I want to highlight how the experience of an uncomfortable chair came into the session through the baby when, crying, he shows us his desire to change position.

The mother was able to help him, taking the baby out of his seat, but in this way she started to experience in her body something uncomfortable.

My suggestion to change the couch with a more comfortable chair will not be accepted not only for the patient's difficulty to accept a new setting but for the reason that the solution doesn't include me and a possible psychological sense for the transformation.

From an analytical point view, the emotional problem concerns all the subjects, and the creative solution of an emotional problem can only arise in the field, in a space where it is impossible to see apart what is of the analyst from what is of the patient.

The baby oriented us to discover primitive emotional elements: through a sensorial experience we can enter the area of primary containment but also the area to be in relation through the body, the movements, the tonicity, the posture.[18]

So, the search for comfort can be seen as a primary unconscious creative quality in the relationship.

The endless effort to find comfort in an uncomfortable chair

For a long time we have distinguished the right tools to psychotherapy from the ones to psychoanalysis using to get this distinction the quality of interpretation and the use of the setting.

In the light of the conceptual developments that have moved the device from an external element of the setting process to a particular arrangement of the minds at work, this distinction has lost some of its value. The concept of comfort in its value of descriptor of a set of variables of the psychophysical relationship between analyst and patient can be a useful tool for taking a different perspective from which to view the therapeutic experience at both high and low frequencies.

These variables help to give substance to the concept of comfort, with the relationship of mind and body of the patient, the analyst and the way they meet in the session.

The convenience that also includes the reality of where you sit, and how often you use that chair or the bed, has an important role in the type of psychic transformations that can take place.

It can be assumed that the analytical instruments, the frequency and use of the chair or cough, contribute to the quality of the experience but do not have a prominent place in generating emotional unison in K or in O and in psychical intimacy that are at the heart of the transformations.

The concept of comfort, just for the fact of describing a complex experience, is a term that opens the contact and the sharing of different points of view. It can only remain in power with the inherent discomfort that permeates what is changing and that relentlessly bends comfort in an experience of discomfort. As Bion wrote:

> The analytic situation stimulates very primitive feelings . . . It is not therefore, really surprising if one of the pair, and probably both, is aware that the psychoanalytic raft, to which they cling, in the consulting room, beautifully disguised, of course, with comfortable chairs and every modern convenience – is nerveless a very precarious raft in a tumultuous sea.[19]

The search for comfort in an uncomfortable chair is therefore the endless effort of analysis and the transformational processes that help determine it.

Notes

1 Domus n. 202, p. 24.
2 Bion 1977.
3 Kernberg IJPA 1999, pp. 1075–1091, tried to point out the specific psychoanalytical features (interpretation, transfer and technical neutrality) and to trace a boundary between psychoanalysis, psychotherapy and supportive psychotherapy with regard to objectives.
4 Alexander et al. 1980.
5 Pasche 2010; Bollas 1979.
6 Neuberger in his contribution to the debate in IJP 1999–2001 wrote provocatively if the length of session or frequency or type of intervention could be seen as more bureaucratic than clinical problems.
7 Brusset 2012.
8 Ogden 1996.
9 Lombardi 2008.
10 Rizzolatti et al. 1996.
11 Children lack the contact with other's people shape. People can change and transform their shapes into "common coin" for relationship. On the contrary autistic children are cut off from the enriching psychological possibilities of everyday life.
12 Bowlby 1979; Stern 2010.
13 Ferro 2008; Grotstein 2007.
14 Bion 1967a, p. 22.
15 Bion 1962b.
16 Bion 1961.
17 Anzieu 1983.
18 Lombardi 2016.
19 Bion 1985, p. 24.

Chapter 9

The Art of Fielding

An analytical field capable of producing transformations is the result of teamwork like that found in team sports, and of a figurative transformation of emotions into dreams, as in an art session. A functioning group of two or more needs to avoid "basic assumption" and remain focused on a work assessment. A good work of art requires the ability of the artist to be himself, to use emotions with authenticity through a process that requires faith and persistence. During his youth, Bion played team sports and throughout his life, he was so inspired by literature and art that at the end of his life, he wrote theory in the form of a novel. In a way, he used his passions to help create a new view of psychoanalysis. Bion bought theoretical tools to manage emotions experienced during analytical sessions as turbulence generated by two or more subjects playing together with words and attempted to transform them into images, metaphors and stories. The analyst isn't engaged in tracing words back to an unconscious message but instead in locating how conscious and unconscious emotions create representations as steps in the transformation of further emotional experiences. Describing the complex unfolding of this process and in particular its necessary basic quality, Bion used the word *truth* to highlight the tension towards the unknown, the absolute not achievable that he named "O". Although he never used the word *authenticity*, it can be hypothesised that this word better describes something close to a subjective active tension towards emotional truth but also something linked to relational experience. This latter allows the transformation of the experience of emotional truth into abilities that are useful in real life. During the analytical dialogue, when an emotion becomes the inner part of a representation, it becomes trapped in a plot, and immediately another idea, imbued with new feeling, pushes one to find another form. How can we know that the forms we are observing in quick succession are authentic forms reaching toward the truth and able to push the creative dyadic process forward? In other words, how can we capture how emotional experience can become an authentic communicative experience? In some ways, the same point of reference can be used to decide the value of a work of art, a complex issue that goes through the history of philosophy, with the further addition that, in the analytic field, the creative dialogue is the result of two subjects' creativity. The issue of how to recognise an authentic form in the psychoanalytic dialogue will be considered only in a limited aspect: the link

DOI: 10.4324/9781003388838-10

between knowledge and aesthetic experience (K↔O in Bion's symbols). One of the first philosophers to recognise the relationship between these two issues was Kant, who theorised that the faculties for aesthetic knowledge are the same ones that the subject uses to discover the world: imagination and intellect. In aesthetic knowledge, these tools aren't directed towards particular facts but contribute to knowledge in a freer way, without a determined purpose, Kant 1781. Bion was inspired by Kant when he described the analytic method to research and explored the achievements of language in the session. He wrote that the two main tools are "speculative imagination" (wild or fantastic thoughts) and "speculative reason", a kind of discipline that we can apply to the first one.[1,2] Through their combined use, the analyst and the patient choose the subject of their conversation, the "selected fact," in Bion's words. But how can the analyst understand how words are effective in feeling transformation?

Outside the field of psychoanalysis, the relationship between knowledge and aesthetic experience has evolved through different philosophers' theories over the last century. Dewey, an American intellectual, described the aesthetic experience as the fulfilment or the condition of each experience. In his opinion, whenever the meanings contained in a weak and fragmented way in common experiences are clarified and focused, every time an experience is actually complete, we are then faced with an aesthetic experience. In Bion's thinking, two ways of discovering psychic reality are always present and in oscillation during the whole creative construction of analytic dialogue: K (knowledge) as a more cognitive experience and O as a transcendental one; the aesthetic form contained in both is able not only to push the process forward toward the unknown, new ideas and feelings, but also to represent a step in which the couple creates the reciprocal experience of fullness. Fullness may be considered part of an authentic way to build experience together, and at the cross-roads of psychoanalysis and aesthetic experience, authenticity appears as a broader concept of emotional truth; it is a word that includes something about style and the ability to reach a sense of contentment and sharing together.

Like the concept of beauty, authenticity refers to a subjective experience, but at the same time it needs to be shared with an other. Therefore, it can be argued that authenticity isn't a concept but rather an experience, oscillating between action and receptivity, not strictly linked with niceness.[3] This way to consider authenticity goes through the form, not just the content, of language; a form capable of arousing surprise, wonder and transformation of the gaze. Next we explore the meaning of authenticity in the context of choosing words in the analytic dialogue.

Playing defence versus the art of building a creative field

The Italian translation of the book title *The Art of Fielding* is *Playing Defence*. Perhaps the reason for a non-literal translation is due to the low popularity of baseball and its rules in this country. In some way this fact allows consideration of how, during the session as a time of playing, the analyst and the patient can oscillate between building a true creative playing field or defending one's own position without living a real experience of creative playing and aesthetic experience. In the co-creation of meaning and dreaming in the space of the session, language and the "body in the language" (the tone, the volume of the voice, the pace of speech) are critical to and inseparable from the life of the ideas. In opposition to the objectivistic point of view, in which efficacy was a quality of the analyst's interpretation, in present thinking the key to efficacy is the subject's relationship with himself, triggered by the relationship with the other. In contrast to the past, in which the analyst paid careful attention not to reveal anything personal, authentic subjectivity, useful for creating a generative field, requires a capacity to use language in a more open way. It is not like self-disclosure but in some ways like an effort to re-create an aesthetic experience, such as reading poetry or listening to music together. Ogden,[4] in his article "On talking as dreaming", clarified the implication of the change of perspective introduced by Bion and the specific operational consequences of his ideas on language in the session. He rejected his original idea that the analyst's interpretations are a view of one of the subjects on the other and came to the extreme conclusion that changing perspective and improving psychic health are the results of dreaming emotions together. Renouncing playing defence means making language free from a unipersonal point of view and a medical one, and instead putting the motor of transformation in the middle. Dreaming together is like playing together with pleasure, and as Winnicott said, psychoanalysis developed as a highly specialised form of playing in the service of communication with oneself and others. But play is something more than dreaming because it includes real experience. So it can be said that if dreaming is knowing oneself as directly triggered by relations with the other, playing is knowing oneself together the other.[5,6,7]

Learning to speak with authenticity and create a playing field

Going back to the main issue, the meaning of authenticity in analytic dialogue became clearer to me through the words of a patient, or more accurately, through my experience with this patient. The following short report contains some ideas of how to develop a style of efficacious interaction through the effort to be oneself.

The starting point

Patient: I dreamed that you and I were in this room sitting on the carpet. I show you the picture of my ex-boyfriend and you give me permission to hang it on the wall. Suddenly we are in my current boyfriend's room.

I feel well near you but, reflecting on the dream, I feel irritated because . . . You know what's up?

Analyst: No, what's up?

Patient: That in therapy one falls in love with the therapist.

Analyst: To overcome stereotypical ideas, we have to play together on the carpet.

Patient: Yes. But, if that is the goal, why do you continue not to use the "informal you" with me?[8] People in general need more closer relationships.

Analyst: The use of "formal you" makes you feel you are down and I'm up. Probably you are wondering whether I like you as an authentic experience, or whether we are trapped in a theoretical, rigid grid.

Patient: I am thinking that the previous boyfriend wasn't really in love with me. We got together and left each other a lot. And our bodies were not really intimate. He was older than me and probably I expected something more, but I don't know exactly what.

[brief silence]

I remember that my teacher, one I appreciated a lot, said that during an oral examination a student shouldn't only repeat what he had studied in the book, but should add something of his thoughts. Once I said that, in my opinion, Romans were more civilised than Greeks, and not a more primitive people as popular opinion would have it.

She shouted at me and said that I couldn't say something so stupid.

She pushed you to say what you thought, but if it was different from her opinion, she embarrassed you in public.

Analyst: I never considered this possibility. I agree that Roman art is less idealised, sometimes a mix of beauty and brutality. I am thinking of a statue of Minerva I saw some time ago: she was represented as a beautiful woman but also with an angry expression. So she seems to me more human than god. I feel this is a closer representation than with other Greek statues in the museum.

Later, reflecting on this dialogue, I thought about how this patient considers the need for authenticity in a circular way, going step by step to the core of the matter. In the beginning she underlined her need to sit on the same level and to be in intimate contact. She talked about her desire for real love but at the same time her fear of such a feeling. She realised through the description of her previous relationship how her expectations can be delusional, not only in the past but also in the session. In psychoanalysis, there's no experience of real bodily intimacy, and she described her delusion through the discussion of her past boyfriend and my use of language to keep distance between us. She wondered to herself and me how we can stay in the paradox of being in touch and at the same time so distant. So her mind moved towards emotional truth, filled by the hypocrisy of the teacher she criticised. Her mind had found a way to reduce idealisation and to seek in the analyst a witness to her courage. Authenticity, in her mind, is saying what she really thinks, giving up the idea of asymmetric roles, not in the liability of the process but in the analytic game.

After this session, the idea of my grasping at theory and the need to continue to research new ways to speak more authentically lingered in my mind. In particular

I focused my attention on the fact, suggested by the patient, that the enemy of aesthetic experience is neither theory nor practice, but submission to conventions. In her references to the love transference and my use of "formal you", I heard the invitation to follow her in the construction of an experience in which emotion isn't only in the words but in the experience, an aesthetic experience, as I tried to say in the last sentence transcribed earlier, in which in the figure of Minerva contained anger at both.

The patient seems to suggest that the psychoanalytic experience is sometimes like a Greek statue: an idealised form of beauty. Roman art, in her opinion, is actually closer to reality, a mix of beauty and hard emotions. In the analytic setting, the importance lies not in her artistic opinion but in the emotional truth contained in the sentence.

So, at the beginning of the session, I heard her make a request to be on the same level. The emotional work, like a magnet, attracts material if it is on the same level as the patient and is determinant for the construction of an effective experience of sharing. So my response wasn't only a way to agree with her but a way to put myself on the same human level.

This was the starting point of my learning from experience, and after this analytic session I tried to change the quality of my language to prioritise the creation of an emotional connection over the interpretation of content.

Recently with another patient

Patient: Before starting, I would like to ask your opinion about a patient I saw this morning.

The mother, a very aggressive woman, wants me to do clinical exams because she thinks that her son could have brain cancer. The child was in perfect health, and I refused to order examinations. So the mother said that she will choose another doctor.

What do you think?

Analyst: (I feel the huge anger of the patient, but I need time to understand.)

You may not believe it, but I had a very similar case. Sometimes family have not studied scientific theory and they don't feel understood if you use science to explain your point of view; but also a doctor feels bad if she is forced to do something she thinks is wrong. [long silence]

Patient: I was thinking about the message I sent you yesterday.

Analyst: I was thinking the same, as if our minds were speaking in silence.

Patient: [showing happiness] The previous session, I wanted to ask you how your holidays went, but I talked a lot.

Analyst: Well, thank you. But now I am not so well, because I was thinking that I didn't answer your message. When I read it I smiled and then, like a child, I reacted as if you had magically seen my expression. It wasn't a message that needs a real answer, but when we don't receive an answer we become angry.

Patient: Don't worry, it doesn't need an answer.

        Now that my boyfriend is more open with me, I am more calm, but I'm afraid of going back. He doesn't want to speak openly about himself and seems to forget the past. He says that in this way, he is a lucky boy. Sometimes I feel that I have to chew thoughts for him.

Analyst: "To chew thoughts" . . . a nice saying. I agree with you; it is different to digest and to remove emotions.

Patient: I think he loves me for this and I love him because he appreciates my body. I wasn't seen by my parents and so I feel like my body is the wrong part of myself. Now I find myself without anxiety, like in the eye of a storm.

The patient was searching for a conscious point of contact with me (in the beginning, she declared that she had decided to start therapy with me because I am not only a psychoanalyst but also a paediatrician) – on old points of contact in our relationship and inside herself to allow her to speak about an emotive crack that threatened to grow in the mind like a cancer.

When I try to understand and describe the fact from different points of view, I am also describing how our different points of view can produce anger in me and in her. I hypothesise that this first connection allowed her to speak about the real emotional crack. Now after a little hint at our separation during vacation and her not caring about me, she can say openly how I have not taken care of her message.

After this first part of the dialogue, in which both our childhoods are working through the experience of being ignored, we enter into the telling the character of a more open boyfriend – a character that describes the new capacity to chew thoughts and to be in contact.

The surprising fact is that, in the words of the patient, the deepest part of the self is in her body and so through our common occupation as paediatricians, the starting point of the session appears to be an effective creative opening of our personal dialogue.

Like in a novel or in a piece of art, the analyst strives to create a situation in which emotions are contained in the experience, rather than in words. The quantity of emotions in the field has to be optimally regulated: too much overwhelms the capacity to play, while too little makes the relationship arid. The optimal regulation of the intensity of feeling and the subjective quality of the words allows the words to cross the relational field and to be caught by the other subject. The goal for therapy to reach the patient and allow a creative, subjective and full relational experience can be described (or summarised) with the word *authenticity*. So, in few words, we can say that a sentence is authentic when at its end there is an other.

Notes

1 The title is a citation of the novel of Chad Harbach published in 2011. In the novel the expression refers to a particular ability of the main character in the baseball game: an unusual gift for fielding, and at the demanding position of shortstop. In this chapter it refers to the art of building a creative interaction between analyst and patient. The Italian translation of the title of this book is *L'arte di giocare in difesa* (*The Art of Play in Defence*).

2 Bion 1997b.
3 Boccara et al. 2009.
4 Ogden 1997, 1999.
5 Ogden 2007.
6 Winnicott 1971b, p. 41; Ferro 2017.
7 LaFarge 2008; Civitarese 2014.
8 In Italian language there is you singular and you plural.

Chapter 10

The binocular vision of a paediatrician and a psychoanalyst

Being a paediatrician has allowed me to observe many newborn babies alongside "newborn" parents in their respective roles as mothers and fathers. These observations were fundamental to my psychoanalytic training and gave me opportunities to better understand the condition of dependency that an infant experiences while learning to think. Indeed, the development of my observational and reflective skills became inextricably intertwined with those of the people I encountered. In addition, as a paediatrician, I have observed both parent-child interactions and situations of hardship, poverty and chronic illness that affected family relationships in the medium and long term.

Here I describe some situations where I focused on brief interactions, adopting a monocular vision similar to closing one eye to see the detail more clearly. These were moments of contact in which the body and mind of mother and child re-created attunement. I want to show how observation perturbed the relational field and contributed, even if only in part, to direct the process towards either well-being or psychic discomfort. In this sense, the paediatrician's awareness of the dynamics within the relational field plays a crucial role.

The first paediatric check-ups come soon after the great catastrophe of birth when the mother-baby system is still affected by a certain degree of instability. During delivery, the child experiences a reversal in the relationship with the mother's body, in the sense that what was a protective envelope becomes a restraint to overcome. Once in contact with the outside world, the baby has to confront new sensations that inevitably present themselves as threatening and to which he must respond with appropriate sensory adaptations. Re-establishing contact with the maternal body, warmth and protection is the only experience capable of counteracting the indescribable anxiety, close to abandonment, that characterises that catastrophic change called birth. Primordial anxiety, a fear of dying that no child can keep inside, systematically re-emerges in the form of persecutory anxiety every time a change occurs.

To be born to herself as a mother, so too must the postpartum woman go through catastrophic bodily changes and similar anxieties of loss that stand in stark contrast to the symbiosis experienced during pregnancy. Moreover, the mother had to regress to preverbal communicative systems and for a while to renounce the

DOI: 10.4324/9781003388838-11

possibility of being an accessible subject able to manage her own time and relationships with other adults.

Therefore, within the experiential space of a paediatric check-up, it is possible to understand how even slightly stressful situations can reactivate the anguish of helplessness and abandonment in both mother and child. So, I started to find it helpful to imagine a paediatric check-up as an extension of the umbilical cord, a relational field where it is possible to experience how the minds and bodies of all subjects participate and condition the facts – an area in which a transit of waste or oxygen and nourishment is conceivable for each participant. This exchange can transform and influence the observable facts.[1]

While the placenta guarantees separateness and preserves the individuality of mother and fetus, within the umbilical cord, it is difficult to distinguish what belongs to one and what belongs to the other. Moreover, a recent study has demonstrated that cells of the fetus can cross the placenta, circulate in the mother's blood and integrate themselves within several maternal organs, building chimeric zones. Something like this happens during an analytic session: there are two subjects with their individuality, but the exchange creates both a whole and a chimeric zone.

I explore these considerations by offering three vignettes from my practice: all three illustrate the impossibility of untangling the contributions of the subjects participating in the relationship.

Mohamed: mirror reactions

Mohamed was born at term and is being breastfed. His parents are foreigners without residence permits. Mohamed's mother speaks very little Italian, and for this reason, she has brought along a friend for support.

Even though I invite her to pick up the baby, she wants me to carry him from the baby carriage to the scales. Once Mohamed is placed on the slightly oscillating plate of the scales, he becomes very agitated. Then, after a startled reaction, we observe the opening of his arms and the stretching of his legs, followed by a sort pulling in and clutching motion (Moro's reflex). Finally, Mohamed starts to cry, and his mother's body does something similar to her baby's: she opens her arms in a gesture of fright and looks towards her friend.

The swinging motion of the weighing scales gives the baby an experience of instability that activates the fear of falling. On the contrary, both the firm surface of the medical table and his mother's arms support the infant's back securely, as it was in the womb, giving him a feeling of safety. In my experience, mothers know how physical fear gets mixed up with bodily sensation and instinctively try to protect the baby. They put the idea of interfering with the objective fact of weight on the back burner and place their hand on the baby's body to protect him or her from the disturbing experience.

Sometimes they comment: "He's crying because he's afraid of falling!" or "He's upset because the scale plate is cold."

Even if the baby is protected from the cold, mothers capture the essence of the emotional experience and delay the medical need by a few minutes.

In Mohamed's case, however, his family's situation of social marginality creates a more significant imbalance of power between doctor and mother than usual. I realise that the mother's refusal to carry her baby to the scales was the first act of submission or deference to someone deemed more capable.

At play at this delicate point is the choice between a more medical relational paradigm, centred on dissymmetry or the possibility of contact that contemplates a diversity of knowledge but not power.

Monica: the umbilical cord

Monica is one week old. She arrives with her mother and maternal grandparents, who systematically answer in the place of their daughter, a severely obese young woman.

I begin to feel irritated, invaded and prevaricated.

They all seem obsessed with food, with the amount of milk Monica takes in, which is considered insufficient even if her growth suggests otherwise. Artificial feeding provides them with an objective measure of the amount of milk the baby consumes.

I am unable to contain the barrage of doubts and questions that they put to me. Grandma replaces the mother in every gesture of care.

I feel myself wanting the examination to end, and as soon as they leave, I open the windows to respond to a physical sensation of air hunger.

It is only after several encounters that I understand that this young woman does not have a partner and has filled in the baby's clinical record with the name of a man who disappeared soon after the baby's conception.

Throughout her pregnancy, Monica tried to emancipate herself and escape from the suffocating bond with her family.

I think back to our first meeting, where I experienced a sense of physical suffocation. I think of the experience of when the umbilical cord is knotted around a baby's neck, cutting off the flow of oxygen and nourishment. Around whose neck did this cord tighten? Probably around the necks of all of us meeting periodically to talk about Monica's development.

Each of us conveys our own needs and feelings of suffocation through the child.

In their excessive and overbearing zeal to care, even the grandparents may be expressing the desire for a life unburdened by a parental caregiving function.

I wonder what I can do to make the situation less asphyxiated? How to attenuate the mother's projection of her chronic hunger for self-growth-promoting relationships into Monica.

For a long time, I have had no idea and taken no initiative; there is only a desire to escape.

Federico: between life and death

Two years before, Federico's mother lost her baby girl to intrauterine suffocation in the eighth month of pregnancy.

At the first check-up, amidst tears, she tells me that she is happy that this new child is a boy like her first one as if gender might create a sort of safe distance from her tragic memories.

In the first few months, she is a very anxious mother. Even if this seems entirely understandable to me, as the months go by, it becomes difficult to be called or urged to respond to messages and emails on an almost daily basis. The more I call upon myself to understand, the more the phenomenon seems to make me experience an unconfessable desire not to answer. Then I receive the following message:

"Doctor, as a woman, only you can understand."

It is a message that tears my being a doctor away from a neutral understanding. I can only understand as a woman, and as a woman I can both feel suffocated by her messages and return the experience of not shirking and, therefore, not dying.

This thought oxygenates me, but how can I give her back something that can also be oxygen for her? How can I give life back to a child who was never born?

I think of Oriana Fallaci's book and how this writer turns the question upside down in the painful story of her miscarriage. She does not ask whether she wants the child, but whether or not the child wanted to live in a harsh world, full of wars, pollution and injustices of all kinds.[2]

I do not know how to do it, and the conscious process stops.

Like something that has continued to flow underground, during a check-up a few months later, I call the child Federica instead of Federico. The mother looks at me questioningly. I told her that her unborn baby was on my mind, and so I made a mistake. I am unable to evaluate the consequences of my slip of the tongue and my explanation. They came out suddenly without adequate reflection. As soon as I recover my attention, the idea of having merged the name of the dead child and the beautiful living child distresses me. Nevertheless, I have done something that the mother has also done in part and that Federico will feel even without being aware of it.

A very long silence follows, and, in my mind, I turn to this unborn child, asking her to help us from wherever she is.

We remain speechless, immersed in the same water, in an understanding that unites us and perhaps constitutes the essence of the primary feminine.[3]

Analytic therapy: who gives birth to whom?

For a physician, birth is an event that involves a woman and a baby in a catastrophic change.

But what does it mean to a psychoanalyst? As the beginning of something new, the concept of birth involves at least two subjects whose existence implies and transforms the other. But unfortunately, there is no conceptual trace of it either in philosophy or psychoanalysis until the middle of the 20th century.

Since the starting period, psychoanalysis considered the birth of the mind from the body and their relationship during life. But, despite that, it has belatedly recognised psychic birth as a phenomenon involving at least two subjects and their mutual interdependence.

Freud developed his theory at the beginning of the 20th century, in a society where power was predominantly male, and women were subjects who lacked "something". Only the birth of a male could give women the fullness that their genitals lacked. A theoretical representation comparable to Gustave Courbet's 1898 painting: *The Origin of the World* depicting a nude woman, supine with her genitals in the foreground, a detail that made critics define the work as pornographic. Compared to other nudes that changed the history of art, this one is unique because the model is faceless: she is not a subject but an anonymous woman who agrees to pose to satisfy the erotic desire of her man, commissioner of the painting.

Immersed in this type of culture, Freud could only imagine the birth of the mind as a progressive development that passes through different stages, all of which are internal to the subject and have as their fulcrum the overcoming of rivalry with the father, the only person considered a real subject.

It would take about 50 years for a psychoanalyst to claim that being born from a woman is a biological but also a psychic fact. Karen Horney was the first to disagree with the Freudian theory that placed penis envy and the repression of libido at the centre of female psychic development and as the engine of neurosis. Instead, she overturned the paradigm and theorised that both men and women envy the uterus as the primordial place of the power to generate and give birth. Horney developed what Melanie Klein first theorised about the creative power of the mother. She was responsible for two radical changes in viewpoints: the discovery of a pre-Oedipal development phase and the equating of play with dreams. In the pre-Oedipal stage, Klein explored unconscious fantasies. They arise from intense bodily exchanges that come before words. She also introduced through equating play with dreams the idea of a creative dialogue between inside and outside.[4]

Winnicott picked up and developed these insights by positing the relationship with the mother as the necessary experience through which the psyche sets up in the body.

Bion took a further step in describing psychic birth as a process in which it is impossible to untangle whether it is the child or the mother who produces it. He theorised the role of the relationship with the maternal mind as the place from which to take his cue to describe some phenomena observable in the analytic relationship in which it is impossible to untangle reciprocal conditioning. In particular, the possibility of transforming sensoriality into dreams has its origin in the ability of a mother in love with her child to use her imagination (reverie) to make sense of the distress the child expresses through crying or body movements. Bion imagined the mother as the first container of infant anxieties, but a container that can process and return these anxieties in a more tolerable form. Later Bion expanded the concept of container-contained to describe a dynamic that recursively repeats itself in the analytical relationship.

Bion and Winnicott initiated a progressive extension of the psychoanalytic method. They transformed the analytic treatment from an epistemological exploration to an ontological experience. This last paradigm requires the analyst's willingness not to understand but to be with the patient to feel and sense the unspeakable that inhabits the core of the most severe and disturbing mental suffering. So as Ogden wrote, Bion and Winnicott were the most influential architects of ontological psychoanalysis. Ontological psychoanalysis has to do with being and becoming.[5]

It explores the origin and emergence of ideas, emotions, and narratives as co-created events.

Starting from paediatric experience, I attempt to explore some of the characteristic features of birth from a psychoanalytic perspective: the sudden loss of a previous arrangement, dependence and regression. Moreover, I intend to investigate what kind of link there may be between these aspects and the feminine.

Birth: too fast a process for the mind

The change of state that characterises birth takes place quickly, as the changes in a natural disaster. Biologically, in the continuity with the maternal body, the baby can face unknown stimuli that could overwhelm its adaptive capacities.

Similarly, the mother must face a sudden loss and mourn this separation immediately after that, a feat she accomplishes by engaging her mind. Thus, it is not by chance that women find themselves in a state of psychic fragility in the postpartum period and are most at risk of breakdown.

At any age, the human mind struggles to adapt to rapid changes to which it initially reacts by setting up primordial defence mechanisms. The subsequent adaptation to change is a process that takes time and, above all, is nurtured by contact with the other; the construction of a new relationship is one of the most influential factors in guaranteeing the evolution of the process and in avoiding defensive sclerotisation.

In this sense, the mutual dependence between mother and child is essential, as evidenced by the difficulties experienced by mothers and babies separated at birth due to prematurity or maternal mental health issues.

Transposed into analytic therapy, one can affirm that it is crucial to consider primordial needs and maintain emotional attunement, especially when transformations imply essential changes in psychic structure. In this core of mutual dependence, we can place the development of some of the concepts and transformations of technique that characterise post-Bionian field theory.

First, field theory is a relational theory, but it also considers intersubjectivity as a structural datum more than others. In this perspective, analytical relationships reflect an interdependence that, as in pregnancy, is impossible to attribute to one or the other of the two subjects.

It is also necessary to clarify that as mother and child are not a dyad, neither are the analyst and patient. Each subject includes a group that can produce well-being or malaise depending on the capacity to reflect upon and possibly regulate the oscillation.

The biological experience of birth allows us to understand how each subject emerges from and into a physical, linguistic, cultural background.

In the small family group, the child is the least able to transform negative emotions; in the analytic situation, there is an infantile analogue urging for change, a proto-mental matrix from which proto-mental phenomena originate (emotional states are an expression).

When these phenomena start to transform, the unconscious emotional climate of consonance (O) is aroused, and shared emotions can grow.

To give an example through events early in life, one can observe how the birth of a child can put the whole family relational system in crisis. In a moment of catastrophic change, couples struggle to manage the emotions that the new relationship solicits and experience what Bion calls the proto-mental, a primitive stage, where discrimination is not yet defined.

The group proto-mental system can evolve towards containment, elaboration and growth or, on the contrary, towards the reinforcement of the cancerous-like development of the "adrenal-attack-escape", "gonadic-coupling", "prolactin-dependence" quotas of the group's proto-mental system.[6]

Something similar happens in analysis: there are moments of expected growth and others when more catastrophic transformations occur. At times such as these, the analyst's ability to manage emotions may or not contribute to avoiding fractures and allowing new birth.

Regression

Freud classified regression as an unconscious defence mechanism. He hypothesised that regression was a phenomenon that returned both children and adults to an earlier stage of development. He further hypothesised that the psychopathology of neurosis could coincide with fixation points in libido development.

The early psychoanalytic literature described regression as a possibility that the patient may reach primitive states of the self. In this sense, regression is a risky condition and a helpful arrangement for actualising new mental configurations.

It is risky because it can lead back to a non-responsiveness of the object. Regression also means seeking a condition of recognition as a premise for the construction of new bonds.[7]

Within the more classical theoretical paradigm, dependency and regression are words used to describe the patient's condition. However, in the paradigm of post-Bionian psychoanalysis, not only it is impossible to disentangle them but also to attribute them to one of the two subjects. The mutual dependence that pushes one to engage in the process of mourning a previous arrangement and the ability to regress within oneself to a language that adapts to the other are intimately interconnected phenomena.

If regression and mutual research between analyst and patient fail, "thoughts without a thinker" – as Bion wrote – materialise in the field. It is similar to the neonatal pathos that gives voice and expression to the proto-mental. It is the responsibility of both analytic subjects to be able to regress to a capacity to detect and accommodate emotions in the belief that what is describable in terms of affections is at the same time a set of cognitive processes.[8]

So the word *regression* in post-Bionian field theory can no longer describe the patients themselves, it can indicate the joint effort to reach areas where the proto-mental can be explored and made to evolve. Attunement is the starting and ending point of this research.

The concept of listening to the patient's responses guided therapeutic practice to carefully consider the patient's ability to tolerate transformative processes and find what we now call sustainable psychoanalysis.[9]

Field theory has added something to the need to focus on emotional attunement description as it can be reached through an aesthetic sensibility. Focusing on aesthetic features allows analyst and patient not only to reach the same emotional place but to reach together a proto-mental state, the basic level from which emotions originate.

I describe three short vignettes. Through them we can learn from the birth experience with its correlates of mutual dependence and how we can find emotional attunement even if we speak different languages.

The silences, the stumbles, the accelerations and decelerations, the repetitions, the redundancies become in this process aesthetic moments of mutual learning. They are the background music, the nonverbal that characterises the search for attunement.

Matilde: a stumbling block

For years Matilde has described her husband as a controlling person. In addition to her husband, I often thought that Matilde referred to the analytic experience that imposes a regularity that is inflexible to personal needs.

By mistake, she received the bill I charged her for one session less at the end of the month. Unfortunately, Matilde made the bank transfer without noticing my mistake.

The following month, however, she did notice it, and as soon as she lay down on the couch, she said in a festive tone:

Matilde: Thank you, doctor! I only saw today when I made the new transfer that you hadn't charged me for the session I missed when I had to go to the hospital last month. I wanted to thank you for that. I always thought that this business of paying for missed sessions was a rigid and somewhat sadistic aspect of analysis, and this time I have to change my mind. I also appreciated that you didn't tell me anything so as not to brag about it.

After such a premise, it is impossible to say that it happened by mistake. However, I feel guilty for being praised for merit that I don't have, and I wonder how to preserve the old rules of payment and this new policy that Matilde is celebrating as if it were a new birth.

Matilde: I have to say that after the scare I had when I thought I had an autoimmune disease, my husband has also been gentler, and we have gotten a little closer. We felt happy to be healthy, and last night we went out for an aperitif after a long time.

I remember that towards the end of my analysis, I asked my analyst if I had to pay him for the two missed sessions while I was in the hospital with my son, who had a suspected bone tumour, and he replied: "Of course, yes".

Fortunately, as for Matilde, the diagnosis had been less severe. While today I can think that the answer might have been methodologically correct, at the time, it had caused a wound, a feeling of distance from the drama I was experiencing. That answer was a sudden and painful fall compared to the help that he had previously given me in this matter.

Matilde had allowed me to repair my old wound in the sense that this memory made me feel very close to her feelings, and what I had unconsciously done gave me the satisfaction (even if false) of being better than my analyst.

This story led me to a point where my ability to manage my emotions and the possibility of being an analyst was in crisis. Yet it was as if I had found myself holding a small and needy part of me that Matilde was taking care of in that absurd way mothers talk to their children when they attribute to the child the achievement of their own needs. So, for example, they say, "You did great! You slept so much because you understood that I needed to rest!"

While it is not rational, it occurs in the relation in moments marked by a strong idealisation of the other, as in falling in love.

Even if the verbal exchange between Matilde and me was a misunderstanding, something happened. We were both happy to share that moment and feel various rigidities transformed without the temporal order of things or the attribution to a particular subject hindering the shared feeling too much.

Matilde had given birth to a less rigid analyst, and whether it was me, my analyst within me or her husband mattered little. What we felt in unison was the contentment and surprise at what had happened.

Antonio: the invention of a couple

Antonio: Doctor, don't you think I was unlucky to leave my girlfriend just before the pandemic broke out?

I haven't met anyone all this year; how can I find another girl? And now everyone can make love freely because couples can meet each other again while I'm about to go crazy: I study and see naked women everywhere. It's torture!

I have to smile and think about Fellini's drawings of his dreams, often with an ironic erotic element.

Analyst: Fellini drew his dreams, and maybe you can too. Who knows, perhaps when these girls are on paper, they will start an adventure.

Antonio: I have never told you about it before, but I love Manga, and I try to draw them a little. To tell you the truth, the erotic ones are not my favourites because when I bought them, they made me feel like a loser. The drawing is different, though.

Analyst: Yes, it is different.

Antonio: Until now, the only way I can get back to my studies is to go to the bathroom and masturbate. If I don't, I really can't concentrate anymore. I will try, as you say, to make a sketch.

   He notices the double meaning of the word "sketch" in Italian connotating both a rough drawing and ejaculation, and bursts into a loud laugh that I join in.

Analyst: It is as if a new couple has been born on paper.

And that is also what happened between us as an analytic couple when we enjoyed a moment of somewhat eroticised but ethically rigorous contact. So, a paradox gave rise to a more playful area in which the isolation and separation caused by the pandemic were upturned.

This vignette also illustrates how the L component (love) is a critical ingredient that Bion made explicit as an essential component for the function of reverie. Still, emotionally the important part of any transformation is the birth of the third, be it a child, a new relational arrangement or an idea.

Nicola: the beginning of kindergarten

Nicola is not settling into nursery school: every morning, he despairs and vomits. The parents ask for psychological support.

The mother has a heart condition and will soon have to undergo major surgery. Probably in the separation that attending school implies, the anxieties of the mother and the child merge and those of the father who, although he does not make it explicit, fears for his wife's life.

The consultation followed by mother-child therapy should help them to metabolise the anguish of mutual loss. Nicola played with pots for many sessions, always spilling the liquid or solid contents onto the floor. His action seems to be very communicative and close to the symptom he has tried to share with his parents: evacuation of the excessive emotional turbulence through vomiting. Although this seems plausible, the interventions aimed at transforming and evolving the game were ineffective. Nicola continued to "vomit" the contents of the pots on the floor, taking particular pleasure in spilling water or small pieces of paper and scattering them with his feet.

When Nicola leaves, it takes me some time to tidy up, dry and retrieve all the tiny bits of paper that have gotten everywhere. Inwardly, I share a certain sense of exasperation with Mom.

As I tidy up at the end of a session, perhaps to curb the difficulty I am experiencing, I fantasise that water and bits of paper are the fluid and corpuscular components of blood and my floor the extension of the body. This fantasy does not lessen my difficulty tidying up, but I feel less irritated in the following sessions. A sense of tenderness gradually appears as if unconsciously Nicola wanted to help his mother by making a heart pump work at its best, capable of reaching even the most peripheral body districts.

Of course all this is only in my mind, but the transformation of my emotions changes the relational climate. When Nicola unfailingly overturns everything, I think of the regularity of the heartbeat that spills the contents of the ventricle into the bloodstream, and I think of how it might be for a child when he feels the mother's anguish and the prospect of her abandoning him forever.

Then I introduce a variation in the game.

When Nicola turns everything upside down on the floor, I join in the spreading of it and invite his mother to do it with me. Once over the initial perplexity, we adults also enjoyed this somewhat transgressive activity, transforming an apparent provocation into a game. Once this first phase is over, I tell them that all the water and the pieces of paper feel lonely and sad and want to get back together, and with my hands, I try to gather everything together. We repeat this sequence a few times, and at the end, I have a pile of paper pulp in my hands that I press a little until it forms a ball, in my imagination, a small paper sculpture of a heart.

The next time we make the ball with water and paper on the table without going through the flooding of the floor.

Jago, a talented young sculptor, fused rigidity and movement by sculpting a series of 30 hearts, each rotating on its axis, displayed in a row to re-create the correct sequence activity. He then filmed these sculptures, achieving the impossible: ceramics that move.

I think Nicola gave life to a creative process because the intersubjective unconscious field could welcome it.

Within a few sessions, Nicola became interested in a new game. I share some thoughts about this transformation with his mother, and I tell her that Nicola has learned to play and is perhaps ready to play with other children. The mother confides to me that joining in the mess-making (spreading water and paper all over the floor) was fun for her and has made the disaster she envisions when she thinks of the operation less frightening. She told me how she was scared of the thought of her blood flowing outside of her body during surgery. Her confiding this detail makes the transformation of the floor into a body make more sense.

In the sequence described, I would like to emphasise that even though transformation occurs through the contributions made by adults, the child is unconsciously connected to his mother more powerfully and effectively than the psychoanalyst.

Therefore, my decision to allow him to take the lead and trust that he was the most capable of unconsciously heading towards life may have been an essential guiding factor in this case.

His mother's operation was successful, and Nicola is now attending preschool.

Where transformation starts

Physical birth is inevitably associated with feelings of intense participation and emotion. Something similar happens when you observe relational sequences between mother and child in which you can sense that you are witnessing, as Winnicott's puts it, "the indwelling of the mind in the body".[10] Although the psychoanalytic theory has drawn much from the observations of mother-baby interactions, much remains to be thoroughly explored to develop new practical approaches to reaching the most fragile and suffering minds.

Within the space of a paediatric check-up, the act of observing the relationship, without putting forward theories of knowledge, as the phenomenological method proposes, has allowed me not only to investigate moments of closeness or moments of difficulty between mother and child but also to see how an experience of contact can set in motion a transformation. Sometimes it is between mother and child in my presence, as in the first clinical case, and at other times it is between parts of myself in my role as doctor or as a product of the group as illustrated by the other two cases.

Suppose we compare these moments of unison to the exchange within the umbilical cord. In that case, intuitively, we can grasp that even if the metabolic function is dislocated outside of one's own being, the subjects who participate in the relationship have the experience of receiving oxygen and nourishment and of being able to deposit emotional waste outside of themselves.

Therefore, what better place to observe and become more aware of the complex dynamics within family-child relationships than in a paediatric outpatient clinic or in mother-baby observation?

It can be observed that soon after birth, both mother and baby have a sort of heightened emotional permeability that allows a third party to experience how it enters the system and introduces elements that affect its evolution.

Some of these observations have partly contributed to my choice of post-Bionian field theory as my primary reference theory.

This theory places considerable value on observations of the primary relationship and explores the psychic birth.

In physical birth as in psychic birth, there are two subjects in relation to each other in which emotions are intertwined and impossible to attribute to one or the other.

Psychic birth, as the final event of a transformation, is a process that, although preceded by a period of co-construction, takes place in a relatively short time. Therefore, it represents, like physical birth, a point of discontinuity with a previous mode of being for the patient and the analyst too. Since rapid transformation generates intense anguish, it requires that the analyst quickly reach the proto-mental place from which it springs. In this sense, regression becomes a shared fact between analyst and patient and not only a backward slide of the patient. Regression is a process of return to an archaic, infantile matrix in which the dependence on the other is radical, and the contact between the minds plays a crucial role.

The bewilderment experienced during this process by both subjects participating in it is the analogue of the struggle between the body of the child and that of the mother during labour.

The first clinical vignette (Matilde) illustrates how this process of re-attunement seems unrelated to what is happening and goes beyond measurable time to tap into a dimension of oneiric temporality.

Antonio's case highlights the erotic aspect of birth. It describes how the analytic couple transformed an experience of loneliness and relative separation into a playful moment of erotic mental unison.

Nicola's case shows how the analytic relationship, as every creative process, involves more than two subjects. In the mother-child treatment, the child is designed as the more fragile subject and often embodies the symptoms. On the other side the child is the subject able to push the others towards the proto-mental part of the field and promote its transformation.

We can say that field theory puts analyst and patient in a place where transformation starts, where the two subjects are on the same unconscious level, and describes better than other theories that the possibility of evolving depends on the capacity to create an emotional unison.

Notes

1 We can never know the facts and truth; we can only partially know when embodied in a narrative, not always verbal, that flows from the relationship.
2 Letter to a Child Never Born, Rizzoli 1975.
3 Winnicott 1971b.
4 Horney 1942; Klein 1932, 1955.
5 Eshel 2017, 2019; Ogden 2017, 2019.
6 Bion 1961.
7 Winnicott 1971c, p. 192.
8 Bion 1962b, 1963, 1965, 1970.
9 Ferro 2011; Collovà 2007.
10 Winnicott 2017d, pp. 139–142.

Chapter 11

Binocular group vision

A method to explore the less accessible areas of the mind

Starting with the body

Vision is a tool for acquiring knowledge, and yet it is the least developed sense at birth. In the first year of life, the activation of cortical areas integrating sight, emotions and the emerging experience of the relationship with the mother makes vision a cornerstone of the relationship with the other and the world. Thus, binocular vision, which reaches full development at around 18 months, is a perceptual event of great importance because it allows the baby to focus on details, be aware of a specific portion of space and its depth and use vision to finalise action. At the same time, it is an event that coincides with the development of knowledge, awareness and ideas.[1] I have seen; therefore, I know. Transposing this premise within the analytical relationship, what does it mean to see, focus, be aware of what is happening in a specific portion of space, and know how to use this information? Since its inception, psychoanalysis has postulated the existence of an invisible plot that conditions choices and relationships. However, the very idea of the unconscious has changed over the last century and consequently, so has the method of exploring those facts that escape immediate comprehension or are entirely inconsistent with a logic of pleasure or convenience.

The inaccessible state of the mind

How can we intuit the unconscious web of relational ties and symptoms?[2]

Bionian theory has as its founding element the assumption that thought cannot be a fact of the single subject's internal world but is ontologically relational. Just as two eyes are needed to see stereoscopically, so two subjects are needed to think. Thinking is possible if one activates the capacity to transform the sensations and proto-emotions (beta elements) that make up the infant's initial bodily sensations into dreams. They become accurate perceptions, i.e. perceptions that have meaning, only by passing through the transformative capacity of another (alpha function), which thinks them up and returns them "digested". Therefore, there is an actual reversal of perspective, whereby it is no longer the unconscious that produces the dream but the dream that produces the unconscious. Conscious and unconscious then become the product of a progressive differentiation operated by

DOI: 10.4324/9781003388838-12

the alpha function "which, giving rise to alpha elements, builds a contact barrier"[3] which marks the point of separation and generates the distinction between them. Bion introduced the term "binocular vision" to describe this relationship between the conscious and unconscious as parts of mental functioning that are different and simultaneously communicating with each other.[4] Although being able to keep them separate is a psychic necessity that prevents psychotic drift, their partial communication guarantees the input of irrational but also creative aspects into cognitive functioning. The contact barrier, the result of a function in a continuous process of formation, can be likened to the function of visual coordination that guarantees the focusing of the image. Beyond conscious and unconscious mental states, Bion in 1997 postulates the existence of a third state of mind that he calls "inaccessible". He refers to proto-mental states as vestiges of physical events experienced by the foetus or in perinatal life, thalamic or subthalamic fears that never had access to processing.

Bion wrote:

I am suggesting that besides the conscious and unconscious states of mind, there can be another one. The nearest I can get to giving it a provisional title is *inaccessible* state of mind. It may become inaccessible because the foetus gets rid of it as soon as it can. Whether it is an awareness of its heartbeat, or an awareness of feeling terror, of sound, or of sight – the kind of sight experienced through the pressure on the optic pits by changes of pressure in the intra-uterine-fluid – all that may never have been what we would call either conscious or unconscious. It is difficult to contemplate because when we are contemplating it, we are in a conscious state of mind – like waking up and saying we had a dream.

(Bion 1997b, vol. 10, pp. 197–198)

Inaccessible states concern the lack of containers (♀) rather than the comprehensibility of contents (♂): the foetus is forced to evacuate everything it cannot contain and tolerate.

We now refer to these proto-mental phenomena more extensively by understanding those facts are recorded in a sensory way and do not spontaneously move towards signification. Instead, even after birth, they are forms of procedural, implicit or non-declarative memory and early traumas that are deposited in this memory without recollection.

The proto-mental system I visualize as one in which physical and psychological or mental are undifferentiated. It is a matrix from which spring the phenomena which at first appear – on a psychological level and in the light of psychological investigation – to be discrete feelings only loosely associated with one another. . . . Since it is a level in which physical and mental are undifferentiated, it stands to reason that, when distress from this source manifests itself, it can manifest itself just as well in physical forms as in psychological.

(Bion 1961, vol. 4, p. 177)

Proto-mental states may invade the subject's mind or body in the form of a psychosomatic illness, or they may invade the group and manifest as a basic assumption.

Basic assumptions, which from a relational point of view appear as a poorly evolved mode of functioning, are nevertheless positioned in Bionian thought as an intermediate level between the proto-emotions that inhabit the individual group members and an aggregation of the group's emotions surrounding a task.

> Starting then, at the level of proto-mental events we may say that the group develops until its emotions become expressible in psychological terms. It is at this point that I say the group behaves "as if" it were acting on a basic assumption.
>
> (Bion 1961, vol. 4, p.176)

In other words, the basic assumption would be a more evolved stage of a group that is totally permeated by a proto-mental state; however, the relation proto-mental states→ basic assumptions is not linear but rather as Bion writes, "it is useful to consider these events as links in a circular series".[5]

Bion suggests that:

> It is convenient to think that the basic assumption has been activated by consciously expressed thoughts, at others in strongly stirred emotions, the outcome of proto-mental activity.
>
> (1961, vol. 4, p. 101)

In the complex "circuit" of relations between proto-mental states and basic assumptions, any starting point can be chosen by the therapist who "must decide what description best clarifies the situation".[6]

Maintaining consistency with his theory of thought, Bion hypothesises that this kind of phenomena can also find transformation in the relationship between minds.

> [I]n my opinion the sphere of proto-mental events cannot be understood by reference to the individual alone, and the intelligible field of study for the dynamics of proto-mental events is the individuals met together in a group.
>
> (Bion 1961, vol. 4, p. 103)

In the proto-mental sphere, the individual is part of a system, although at other mental levels he or she has achieved greater individualisation. For example, it is only in a group dimension that it is possible to explore pain signalled through the body.

The network of relationships that make up the proto-mental system is not directly visible; it can become so when this network is ruptured and manifests itself in the suffering of one or more of the group members.

Wild, unstructured, unconnected, often uncomfortable, aggressive and shameful thoughts are how the proto-mental emerges in the group. They are, however, not only the manifestation of a negative but, to some extent, can also be seen as elements awaiting transformation; they continue to circulate until the collective alpha function (a functional analogue of the maternal) makes them thinkable and thus sayable.

In groups, too, it is the trans-individual that thinks, not the individual mind, and it is not by chance that Bion defined the relationship between the subject and the group using the same term used previously to describe the relationship between conscious and unconscious: binocular vision.

Exploring what does not work in the therapeutic relationship

Starting from these shared theoretical premises, a group of psychotherapists took on the task of exploring certain difficult-to-access aspects of our mental states through the methodology which is described later.

The whole day's work is divided into two stages. During the first three hours of work, a participant reads two sessions with a patient the therapist considers as being hard to reach, without making explicit anamnestic or psychopathological data. The difficulty remains an implicit, subjective fact. The presenting therapist may feel that the difficulty lies in the relationship, in the patient's pathology or in the occurrence of demands for settings that are distant from the more established ones. This choice makes it possible to avoid being blinded as far as possible by historical reality and thoughts already thought.

Since the task focuses on analysing the transcription of the dialogue of two sessions, this first part is referred to as the "group session".

This first part is similar to the "weaving thoughts" method described by Norman and Salomonsson in the way of presenting the sessions and the use of free associations by the participants, but it is also characterised by unique features.[7]

The "weaving thoughts" method is inspired by the Bionian postulate that in groups it is possible to realise that thoughts without a thinker can be accepted and formulated more openly. The group in this first phase proceeds by creating associative chains in which a word refers to a thought and a thought to a new word. In addition, images transport the categories of discourse into a visual space that de-saturates them of meaning, creating a new openness to other possible implications.[8]

At the end of the first part the analyst gives feedback to the group putting in evidence how the group thinking had caused difficulties in the therapeutic process in the patient-analyst couple.

The particularity of the method lies in the intersection of the biological model of focusing and the group's attempts to grasp the sense or nonsense of proto-mental states in the relational field.

It is possible to describe processual moments through which associative chains are generated and progressively refined as the group continues to reflect on the dynamics of the therapist/patient and the dynamics within the group itself.

This second part is referred to as "group dynamics".

Three moments can be described by mediating their definition from the physical level:

1   simultaneous perception
2   fusion
3   stereopsis.

Simultaneous perception, in the physiology of biological vision, refers to the ability to simultaneously perceive images presented to both eyes. Transposed to the group, we can identify this level in the mental capacity of each subject to think, that is, to have a reasonable separation and communication between conscious and unconscious. Before being something that concerns reading two different levels of group functioning, binocularity exists within each participant. Each member of the group can make rational comments or say something non-sensical while waiting for that thought to find meaning through the psychic work of the group itself.

Fusion refers to the ability to derive a single visual representation from two similar but not identical retinal images. A prerequisite for the fusion of two eye images into a single one is that the visual directions of the two eyes are similar, i.e. both eyes observe the same area of space, and there are no deviations in the optical axes.

At the level of group functioning, fusion is both a process and a result. The group mind proceeds using the mental coupling of two group subjects. First, the image or thought provided by a member of the group is received by another who creates a space within the mind where differing ideas can coexist. Then, if the receiving subject does not feel invaded or anxious, he or she presents the group with something that is a synthesis of what the subject has received and thought by him- or herself. So, each member of the group creates internally a "binocular vision" that each member offers to the others through a new narrative or symbolic representation. In this case of successful synthesis, when the subject who begins and the subject who follows say something to the group, they are both looking in the same direction and observing the same area of the field represented by the account of the sessions.

When synthesis is unsuccessful, the group registers the phenomenon in terms of discomfort. It is like momentarily seeing double.

Fusion does not mean agreeing but alludes to a process of synthesis that emerges when the confrontation with the other is free from persecutory experiences.

The result of this process is that the group can see how it has come to elaborate on the (implicit) aspects of difficulty that the therapist-patient couple were going through because the group was able to experience and process them.

Stereopsis is the psychic ability to derive information about the depth and spatial position of the object from the minor differences in the retinal images of the two eyes. This function pops up in the mind through integration with cortical functions.

In groups, this process results from thinking and hearing. Every comment is something between subjects and the group's history. It is, therefore, artificial to subdivide the group's work into the working sessions and the group's dynamics. This subdivision has the sole purpose of facilitating the description of a complex process.

Associative work, therefore, always responds to individual and group logic.[9]

At the end of the second part, the analyst gives to the group feedback of the work made, trying to put in evidence how the group dynamic intercepted the difficulties of the therapeutic process of the analyst and the patient at a more complex level.

A short artistic digression

In the lower margin of the last page of his work entitled *Contributions to the Theory of Pictorial Form*, Paul Klee drew a face whose eyes are squinting and very differently shaped.

The left eye has a black, circular pupil, while the right eye is larger and has a vertical, slanted pupil, similar to that of a cat (see Figures 11.1 and 11.2).

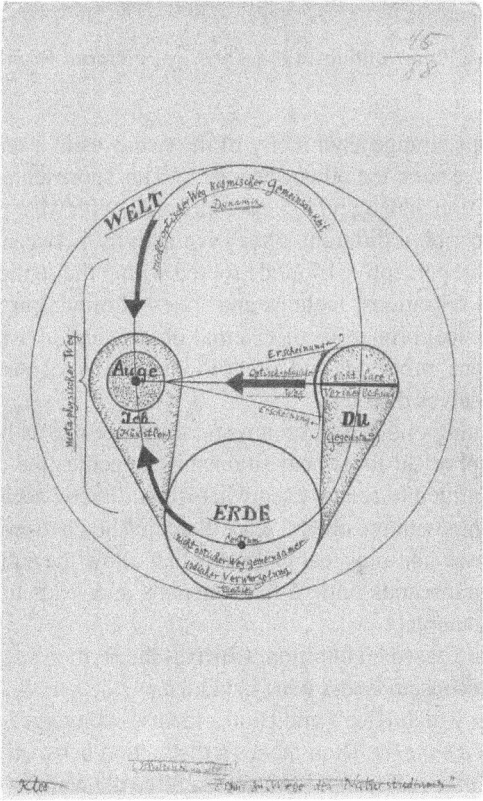

Figure 11.1 P. Klee, *Theory of Pictorial Configuration.*

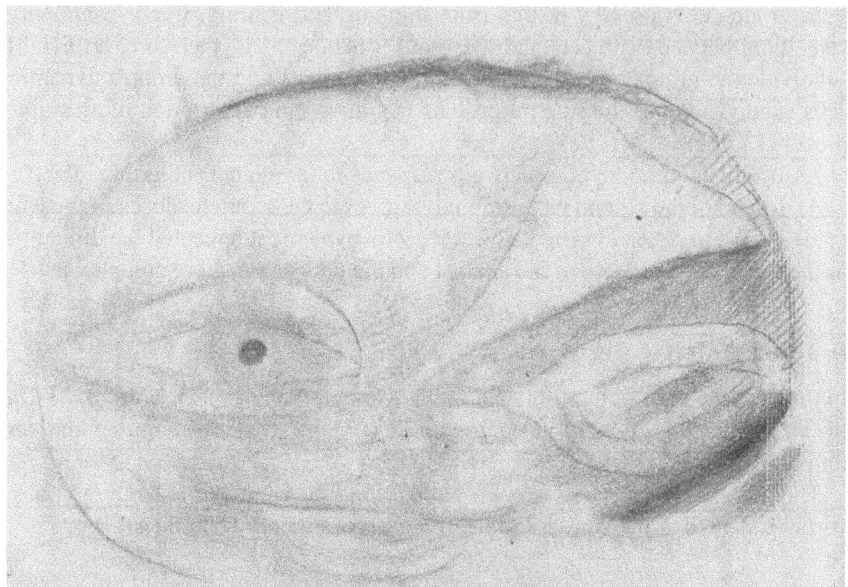

Figure 11.2 P. Klee, *Contribution to the Theory of Pictorial Form.*

Klee clarified the strange asymmetry of the two eyes in a sentence noted in his "Diaries": "One eye sees, the other one hears." This short sentence has the quality of a dazzling intuition, having no logical connection with what precedes or follows it. It does not describe a different perceptive activity between the two eyes, but their more ancestral perceptive bi-mode rooted within the sentient body. What one "hears" generates sensations, feelings and states of mind, but also intuitions that transcend the physical properties of external objects and allow us to be aware of realities, phenomena, processes and connections that do not have the possibility of manifesting themselves directly.

Therefore, defining one eye as seeing and the other one as hearing, rather than indicating a metaphorical functional strabismus, specifies the twofold root of his artistic work committed to seeing even what is not directly accessible to the eye.

In his relationship with the object, Klee distinguished between an optical physical pathway and two non-physical pathways that allow the subject to enter into a relationship that transcends optical fundamentals and leads to what he calls the humanisation of the object.

The two paths are based on intuition, which as the etymon suggests, means to see within, to bring to consciousness what is hidden.

Is this a point at which Klee's and Bion's theories converge?

In *Taming Wild Thoughts*, Bion makes a distinction between speculative imagination and speculative reasoning. Both are useful to the working-through processes of psychological work. We have to keep a rein on speculative reasoning because it can be invasive like weeds. Bion underlined that there is no progress without imagination, even in the natural sciences, and all the more so when dealing with "facts of feeling".

"Speculative imagination" as described by Bion, is a useful tool for exploring the inaccessible part of the mind that is not part of the conscious/unconscious system. It is the space-time between beta and alpha elements, the transitional space between body and mind.

"This case is no coincidence": the interface between group dynamics and the sessions presented

The group experienced stereopsis on becoming aware of an interface between the case presented and the intersubjective dynamics. As an aside, the selection of a patient to present to the group is not only based on the obstacles and challenges of the therapeutic work but also on the basis of the prevailing emotion or dynamic setup that permeated the group in the previous meeting. This observation led one group member to state ironically, "This case is no coincidence!"

The observational process that started in this way produced exciting developments. Paradoxically, each case presented assumes the task of taking care of the group by carrying out the emotional processing of aspects that were undigested or had remained hidden in the previous meeting.

This surprising fact exemplifies what Bion described as the interchange between container and content.

> [There is] an oscillation that at a certain moment places the analyst in unison with the container and the analysand with the content and in the next moment, their roles are reversed.
>
> (Bion 1975, p. 148)

In other words, the group takes care of the therapist-patient pair's difficulties, and the therapist-patient pair takes charge – through the group – of elaborating the dynamics that inhabit it. The fact that the group allows itself to be affected by the prevailing emotions in the clinical account is also an indicator of the group's ability to be in unison with the therapist-patient pair's emotional experience. Before the formalising of any thought, this fact of being in oneness is essential in both the individual and trans-individual therapeutic process. This tension towards "at-one-ment" may also be the matrix of some of the group's difficulties over the years.

Besides, according to Winnicott, the analyst's partial failing is a necessary element in an effective analytic process.[10] For Winnicott, it is only through partial failings on the part of the analyst and the group that it is possible to gain access to areas of unelaborated experience.

The main difficulties in the working group were the exit of two group members at two distinct times and the shift to online meetings during the two years of the pandemic, resulting in a reduction in working time.

These events, which took place over the seven-year period during which the group met, may, in retrospect, also be thought of as events having to do with the attempt to descend into the primitive states of mental functioning. In these circumstances, it became clear that the therapist and the group were not only able to share the patient's feelings but could also be drawn into experiencing the patient's psychic collapse. The collapse may have to do with an amputation that occurs at the relational level before existing in the mind. The group can therefore only reproduce such situations and go through these relational ruptures, which may be reflected upon *a posteriori*.

What has so far been presented in theoretical terms is now illustrated through two examples of the working group's meetings.

First clinical situation

A therapist reads out two sessions to a group of therapists (participants). (The following is a summary of the full content.) What is essential here is to illustrate the emergence of binocular vision at the interface between the functioning of the therapist-patient pair and that of the group.

The first session contains elements of visual fatigue, uncertainty between perception and imagination and the bad feelings elicited by the sense of sight. So, we may think of these phenomena as circulating between patient and therapist as thoughts in search of a shared meaning.

First session

The patient enters the session looking down. "Not well this week, my eyes feel tired, but I don't understand why. I stayed up late last night."[11]

He tells the analyst how he spent the evening with his new partner, Valeria, whom he has been dating since breaking up with his previous girlfriend, Maria. The patient describes this new relationship as very fulfilling, which is why he does not understand his feeling of tiredness. He attempts to explain it by saying that, in addition to being up late the night before, he has been having nightmares that sometimes wake him up in the middle of the night. The therapist notes that his beautiful blue eyes fill with tears, and she offers several reflections that help the patient connect the present moment with painful aspects of his past experience.

The patient then tells the analyst how, as a present for his partner's birthday, he put together a playlist of songs and a collage of photographs accompanied by romantic messages. He speaks of his gesture with pride as if it were a confirmation of his having always felt like "the gift-giving magician".

Then he recounts how he happened to catch a glimpse of his old girlfriend two nights before, while he was in a bar with friends. He ventures that he is not sure if it really was her and wonders if this explains why he did not rush away. He is proud of this reaction because he had explored such an eventuality many times in fantasy and dreams, both of which caused him considerable anxiety. Reality, however, is not as bad as he imagined.

The reading ends with the analyst remarking on the intense exchange of glances with the patient at the end of the session.

Second session

The patient dreams about his previous girlfriend, a nightmare from which he wakes up screaming. When he tells his new partner about the contents of the nightmare and what happened the night before, an argument breaks out that puts the relationship at risk.

The night before, he really had met his previous girlfriend, and there had been a heated argument. He does not remember much of what happened because, shortly after the encounter, he got heavily drunk, and it was his friends who later told him what had happened. Since adolescence, he had been using alcohol to retreat emotionally from any unbearable situation.

The patient had had another violent outburst of rage, like the ones he used to have before starting therapy.

This inability to contain himself continues to be, as it was in the past, a source of great difficulty for him.

The therapist notes, "while he talks to me, I feel the urge to lower my gaze, I feel confused, and I think I am tired too".

Morning: the group of participants works on the relationship between the therapist and patient

Participant: It occurs to me that in his novel *Limonov*, Carrère writes that it is common for young Russians to drink for days until they fall into a sort of ethyl coma.

Participant: I saw a TV series where ghosts were "real" entities. And ghosts do sometimes really exist, as it happened here in the group (referring to the angry outburst of dissatisfaction that sealed one group member's decision to leave). Seeing the ex-girlfriend seems to have triggered something within the patient. That something was registered in the body, also within the therapist in terms of confusion and tiredness.

Participant: So Mary, the first girlfriend embodies something dissociated that is registered in the body more than in the mind.

Participant: How was his relationship with his mother? (The group had established in advance that participants could ask direct questions, which would not be addressed by the therapist but would instead be elaborated by the group.)

Participant: I imagine him as a child being told by his mother, "Why, you're such a gift-giving magician", acknowledging the affection reflected in his little gifts.

Participant: The idea of a magician brings to my mind the omnipotent aspects though which the patient tries to compensate his inferiority feelings but also the image of a rabbit coming out of a hat with a surprise effect. The patient is probably a shy man, like a rabbit, with severe relational difficulties, but the idea of a magician also evokes childhood experiences of playing and of wanting to amaze and be amazed.

Participant: So Maria can be viewed as a character who harbours distinctive aspects of the self that are not acceptable, ghosts, but also free and wild aspects.

Participant: Valeria, the second girlfriend, on the other hand, has a valerian sedative effect on him. The somewhat dull and conformist steadiness of the relationship with Valeria may also reflect that obsessive part that protects him against the unknown and turbulence.

Participant: We should consider that this obsessive part, besides being harmful, allows the patient to hold on to the setting. Being able to build a relationship before it runs into turbulence has an importance.

Participant: Do you know the clothing advertisement that shows an apparently racist slogan on a T-shirt with the intention of getting an anti-discriminatory reaction? "The more hate you wear, the less you care"?

The group discusses the ambiguity of the message. The group then brings up another image by the same clothing brand showing a very elegant woman who is running and holding an unkempt and depressed-looking child by the hand.

The group thinks that these two images represent something that describes the patient on an unconscious level: the premature severance of the maternal bond at the root of his anxiety, and the hatred that emerges violently from time to time in his emotional relationships, echoing that old feeling. The patient was left alone before he was able to deal with that reality and the violent emotions to which it gave rise.

Participant: In order to explore such primitive states of experience with the patient, the therapist would need to open up an area of play with him in which the patient, instead of terror, could experience being surprised by himself. To protect himself, he has chosen to work in the family business, doing a job he does not like which offers comfort and security. He feels the same way about his relationship with Valeria. The group thinks it would be good if therapeutic interventions could help transform Maria from being an excitatory, terrifying experience into a playful one.

Participant: [jokingly] the patient should swing more towards Maria (alluding to Marijuana) than towards Valeria (alluding to Valerian).

Participant: The slogan on the T-shirt is aggressive, whereas he seems to be pretty compliant. After all, the gifts he gives are quite ordinary and unsurprising: even if he does present them as original, they are not exactly "a Christmas tree in July!".

Participant: He should put his rage into song like rappers do. Like Jaz does to the music of De Andrè.

Participant: But coming into contact with Maria is catastrophic, and even the therapist doesn't know what to do with the Maria part.

Participant: Maria needs to be brought into the analytic discourse, but in small doses (again alluding to Marijuana).

Participant: At the beginning, instead of Maria, I had heard Malia: there is desire, seduction, wanting to come into touch with strong emotions, but also a fairly healthy need for dependence that he is unable to achieve.

Participant: A friend of mine was given seeds from Mejugori that turned out to be marijuana seeds. She kept the pot on the stairs and was proud of the way the plant grew, as if it was a miracle related to where it came from. It was a neighbour who told her what it really was.

Participant: Years ago, when I was on holiday in Morocco with a group of friends, we were trying to get away from a car that was following us and we stopped at a campsite that turned out to be a hashish sorting centre. We left a few days later, each carrying a small dose, and then got stopped on the road by the police. Fortunately, the policeman turned out to be in partnership with the fake campsite's owner. So that's how we avoided the horrendous experience of ending up in jail!

The group laughs, and there is a very playful atmosphere.

Participant: In a film I saw recently, it gradually becomes clear that everyday life takes place in an enclosed city. The landscape beyond it has been devastated by a nuclear catastrophe.

The group agrees that what is missing is an intermediate zone between the excitatory experience (Morocco, marijuana and the risk of imprisonment) and the rigid containment within a bubble of apparent normality preserved through splitting. There needs to be an in-between area where experiences can be transformed into play.

Report of the analyst on the work done by the "group session"

In this first phase, the group analyst assumes the task of making the group aware of the transformative work done.

The analyst describes what happened in the margins of the discussion:

- The sessions contain many references to the eyes, and one wonders what relationship this might have with binocular vision.
- At the beginning of the reading, a participant reported having two copies of one page while missing a transcript segment.

These could be a concrete-body transposition of proto-mental phenomena that have hindered the patient's or the therapeutic couple's capacity for symbolisation.

The analyst organises and reports back the group's discussion along two axes: the already consolidated tools for thinking and the more innovative ones.

The group describes how the patient's narrative was organised around the split between Valeria and Maria, two parts of the patient that have been defensively separated. The group's associations also move between two polarities: through very pertinent references, the group inhabits a civilised territory that simultaneously tries to keep out a subhuman part that is the victim of a catastrophe.

The same narrative is expressed more playfully with the allusion to the Maria (marijuana) part, a somewhat drugged but also vital part, and the Valeria (valerian) part, which instead represents the tension towards a defensive sedation of something dangerous and yet also critical.

The group initially follows a more classic approach by using the concept of splitting but then begins to explore how to create an intermediate area where the process of unification can begin.

Starting from the living presence of the ghost of the ex-girlfriend, the group dwells upon how there is a past still living in the present that concerns the patient and the group itself. As with the patient, a participant attempts to manage turbulent emotions by re-establishing a temporal order, referring back to prior events, and creating order in the face of emotionally chaotic situations. That was just what the therapist had done in the session.

In order to move towards a transformation into play, the historical sense of time must be able to fade into the background. As in real child's play, the causal and temporal constraints of reality are not relevant to the psychic processing of painful truths.

At this point, the group searches for a way to identify the factors that can foster this kind of transformation.

Wearing the same T-shirt

The reference to the T-shirt with its publicity campaign slogan increases the group's awareness of the effects of the words "worn" by the therapist and the type of reaction they may elicit. (Some participants found the slogan compelling, while others found it distasteful.)

Moreover, mention of the T-shirt that everyone can wear reawakens the group's awareness of how the patient should not be the only one to experience the difficulties.

The therapist needs to wear the same T-shirt as the patient in order to be in the same emotional place.

Surprising and being surprised

The intermediate space that needs to be opened is gift-like, but we may need to break the stereotype of gifts and be capable of creating something truly surprising. For example, the image of the magician evoked by the patient alludes to a real surprise, to something that disorients, and the group picks up on this with its mention of the rapper who sings to the music of De Andrè or a seed from Mejugorie (a religious pilgrimage destination) that becomes a flourishing marijuana plant.

One participant's personal recollection of his youthful adventure on the border between licit and illicit, fun and possibly tragic consequences seals this transformation.

The protagonist of the escapade shared with the group adds that the name of the campsite in question was Ketama. Picking up on the assonance between the name Ketama and the Italian *che ti ama* (who loves you), the group agrees that a loving psychoanalyst must wear the same shirt as the patient, and wonders why, without slipping into self-disclosure, such an adventure could not be shared with patients, perhaps by starting off with "a friend of mine happened to . . .". It would be way of using narrative to share the difficulty of foreseeing consequences or how in some difficult situations, our defensive behaviours can spiral out of control.

This narrative provided the group with an opportunity not only to discuss the therapeutic factors that can foster a transformation into play but also to experience it. The letting go of pre-packaged categories of thought, moments of shared pleasure and the space to fantasise and to narrate resulted in a shift from a "The patient has a problem" discourse to a "We have a problem" discourse.

Afternoon: the group works on the interaction between the dynamics of the therapeutic couple and the group itself

During the course of the afternoon, the analyst's task is to draw attention to the emotions circulating through the group and how it attempts to process them.

A participant recounts a dream featuring some of the group members. The comments soon come to an end and concern only the concrete description of the type of flower that appears in the dream: the Lunaria. With its disc-shaped translucent seedpods, it looks more like the moon than a flower.

A long silence follows the telling of the dream.

Participant:	But do you think we need the afternoon? For me, it feels artificial to have two separate times because things that affect us as people and as a group also emerge in the morning.
Participant:	In my view, as I have already suggested, we should take the afternoon discussion outside and have a walking meeting.
Participant:	A less rigid use of space . . . I've been doing the same thing with patients' time: I've seen time and again how an abrupt interruption produces a fracture that sometimes we cannot repair.
Participant:	[jokingly] Freud had a dog that "kept time" with his patients by getting up when the analytic hour was up.
Participant:	That reminds me of how once during a trip, we went on this night tour by boat to observe the eyes of crocodiles when they came up to the surface. When light shone on them, the crocodiles just froze like hares in front of car headlights.
Participant:	Hares and crocodiles . . . it's curious how you put two such opposing animals next to each other. Maybe there is something of the hare and the crocodile in us.

Analyst: Perhaps the many references to "looking" in the patient's sessions and the printing mistake that exposed one member of the group to the experience of getting lost and the realisation of having entered a repetitive loop now make sense. At first, the group seems slightly frightened and bewildered as if threatening eyes were about to emerge.

Participant: Perhaps we are split in two like the patient. And then, talking of splitting, I'm reminded of how two people left the group. That's something I still can't swallow.

Participant: Maybe that's why I feel like "walking and talking" outside. It's a sort of middle ground between running away and staying, not a split, a middle ground.

Participant: Of course, splitting is also a way of putting things in order because confusion is a disturbing feeling and it's hard to stay with it. The silence at the start of today helps me to understand something more about my patients' silences.

Participant: The first part of the work feels to me like watching an emotionally engaging film; the second resembles the discussion after the film, to which many in the audience react either by leaving or wanting to do so. Moving from emotional immersion in a story to critical reflection is helpful; it lets us see things we might not otherwise have noticed, but it is also tiring.

Participant: The same must be true for our patients: for both patients and therapists, it's one thing to narrate something, it is quite another to reflect upon it. When there is no playful or narrative atmosphere, we get scared and feel like running away.

Participant: We should also make use of the stories that came to mind this morning with our patients; for example, the one about the seeds from Mejugorie was fantastic.

Participant: I notice now that no one commented on the dream in which N. (a participant) leant out of the boat to pick a Lunaria flower.

Participant: Maybe that's what we're doing now: leaning towards the patient is telling stories, not making interpretations.

Report on the "group dynamic"

Analyst: There may be something that is not easy to reach in the therapeutic relationship or our thinking. After all, our experience was similar to the patient's; his emotions were reproduced and amplified in the group, and we also experienced how difficult it is to hold it together. For example, we verbalised it in our division of the working day into two blocks; the patient voiced it through two characters in his story: Maria and Valeria.

Then Freud's dog emerged. Whether it be true or false, we considered this story to be the expression of the ability to keep time, to keep pace with wants and wishes and the need to set limits. Besides, keeping time with the patient does not just mean telling him when the hour is up but also keeping pace with him, and the afternoon's work also contributed to our understanding of this.

Being a bit of a hare or a crocodile speaks again of the paralysis that dwells within us when we have to find new ways of dealing with fear and aggression. Using "fight or flight" as a way of resolving tension is always present as an instinctive way of functioning.

Lastly, it was from the dream of reaching out to grasp something that this possibility of using our stories and associations in a non-invasive way to expand the field emerged most clearly.

Second clinical situation

The presenting therapist starts by saying:

> The patient and I missed two weeks of sessions due to my commitments; the patient then sent me a text message saying that she could not come for reasons related to her own studies. Before the session I am about to read, she sent another text message to let me know that she would be late.

First session

The therapist reads very fast and intersperses the reading with slightly awkward giggles. She tells the group that this is her attempt to convey the difficulty she is experiencing working with this young woman.

After an awkward giggle the patient says: "I fucked up". She adds that she wrote to the doctor (later understood to be a colleague) who is trying to keep her at a distance. There seems to have been an affective tie with him and recognition on his part of the relational capacities she brought to her work with adolescents, oftentimes being the one to suggest effective solutions in moments of crisis.

(The reading of the therapist is very fragmented, and the group finds it extremely difficult to follow. What does emerge is that the patient works as an educator in a therapeutic school community.)

The therapist cautiously suggests that seeking out the doctor, someone who might to listen to her, may also be related to their long break.

Patient: If he doesn't answer me and doesn't want to show up, then he shouldn't post pictures on Facebook. In one photo, there was a colleague just behind him wearing the same T-shirt as him. I notice certain details.

The patient says she cried for days and then tried to get in touch with the doctor, but this did not help her. Yet previously, he had complimented her on her way with young people while all he is good at is prescribing antibiotics for physical ailments.

She speaks of her relationship with a colleague to whom she first opened up but by whom she then felt judged. She told her that one of her heels was hurting to which the colleague replied that that kind of pain was related to mental rigidity.

Therapist: The doctor was an attempt to have personal contact with someone, but it didn't work out. It is as if you had lost part of me, and a part of you too.

Patient: Yes. You know, I hadn't thought about that. Here I understand things better.

Second session

The patient arrives at the same time as a telephone technician who should have come an hour before and with whom the therapist makes another appointment.

The patient remarks that this is how everything goes in Italy: there is no respect for rules or appointments. Just that day her professor was nowhere to be found during his office hours and so she took the opportunity to study and try to graduate. She goes on to say that thanks to therapy she now feels more able to learn even though studying and working are very tiring.

She also pressed her father to finish the refurbishment of her flat, with none of the usual violent quarrels.

Previous arguments had intensified into throwing things and causing damage to the home.

She talks about visiting a dying uncle who, despite his condition, is happy to see people, whereas there is always such a knife-edge atmosphere in her house. They are constantly reminding her that she needs to lose weight, be less preoccupied with the internet and help out more. In short, they are very intrusive and obnoxious.

Therapist: [implicitly including herself] They touch upon sensitive issues without realising they are causing hurt.

Morning: the group works on the relationship between the therapist and the patient

Participant: Instead of She didn't come for reasons related to her own studies or her suicide. There must be a reason.

Participant: It's challenging to create an intimate space. She is a difficult patient to contain. One would have to breathe her in as we did earlier with the roses.

Participant: The reading speed obviously made it hard to listen and think. I noticed that you slowed your reading down at the part when the patient said, "I notice certain details".

Participant: Maybe we should look for her in the details too.

Participant: The speed of her speech might have something to do with the fact that there was a prolonged interruption; on the other hand, the speed serves to keep her at a distance, as if she were creating a smokescreen.

Participant: Laughing hysterically and talking fast to keep things that are too difficult to say at a distance. The patient also said that she had been unwell, but all in a rush and laughed immediately afterwards.

Participant: Of course, the telephone network technician arriving with her makes us think that some communication problem also exists with the therapist.

Participant: It strikes me that the patient moves around like a ball inside a pinball machine. The pinball machine is a container in which to play. In short, chaos comes to my mind and the search for something to contain it and transform it into play.

Participant: It's as if she were doing a kind of dance to keep in time. She moves closer and farther away as if to find a rhythm.

Participant: It reminds me of children who run hither and thither out of their anxiety.

Participant: I focused on some of the words that describe their communication – the session starts with a text message – then the patient says: "I went on without thinking" – then she adds there were errors in the communication – there are many contradictory messages.

You (addressing the therapist) suggest to her that outside the framework of therapy, in your absence, everything is more chaotic and acted out.

Participant: It reminds me of certain films about attachment featuring dissociated children. It is as if a connection were missing between parts of her and the outside.

Participant: It reminds me of some of Picasso's cubist paintings of asymmetrical faces, a kind of composition of parts.

Participant: On my way to work, I stop off at a bakery where there are two shop assistants, one of whom is more composed, while the other one is always laughing and seems a bit over the top. I used to prefer the quieter assistant but the other day, I noticed that the other one has a deformed hand like a crowbar. It made her being over the top seem less annoying to me.

Participant: We too should see the beauty of this patient, deformity and all.

Participant: In Ogden's book, *Reclaiming Unlived Life*, there is a patient with cerebral palsy. Even Ogden himself had difficulty accepting this patient. Then the patient had a short dream in which – says Ogden's patient – "I was myself, washing the car with the radio on".

Ogden comments that after realising his own difficulty as an analyst in accepting the patient's handicap, the patient has a dream in which he can be himself, do ordinary things and take care of his deformed part as well.

Participant: We all, patients and therapists, feel like fleeing from the monstrous parts of ourselves. It takes time to build up an intimacy that embraces these parts.

[Long silence]

Participant: This long silence feels to me like an incubation time.

Participant: The patient speaks like a rapper. It is hard to understand the words but you get caught up in the rhythm.

Participant: Yes, at the beginning, the therapist asks her, "S., what's happening?" The therapist tries to create a relational framework while she is on the physical level.

Participant: There is often improvisation in rap. What does that mean? What communication tools do we need to hone?

Participant: In rap, there are no exchanges with the audience like there are at a rock concert. On Sunday, I was at a folk dancing festival and there was a courtship dance, where, through imperceptible movements the young people exchanged signals for example indicating that they wanted a date in the evening.

Participant: In actual fact, the patient listens a lot. If you play "the doctor", however, it immediately gives you an overly professional aura. She's the one who wants to reverse the role and teach you something.

Participant: How do we keep relationships alive without getting too close?

The song "Good evening doctor" is evoked in which a lover phones her beloved (the doctor) at home to invite him over. The whole conversation reflects the doctor's inability to answer clearly because he is at home with his wife.

Participant: The film *The Lives of Others* comes to mind. There is an intrusion in the song and the film, not a good kind of closeness.

Participant: She's a patient who has not had any recognition. Sometimes as therapists we do what the doctor did in the song: we say "How are you?" to someone who has called to arrange a tryst.

Participant: Of course, she explodes. She is judgmental about the telecom technician's lateness, but she is also critical of herself. When she cannot accept herself, then all hell breaks loose.

Participant: In the second session, anger emerges in response to psychophysical problems (being overweight, the psychic discomfort of an adolescent who is not understood by the doctor working with her). Perhaps we are the ones who, like the doctor, want to give out antibiotics instead of psychic understanding. Then there is the colleague who tells her that her heel inflammation is a matter of psychic rigidity. Again, it is this lack of recognition that makes her angry.

Participant: Sara, "Sarà" means will be (in Italian) (uncertainly). I want to be understood now!!!

Participant: There are organisms called extremophiles that are able to withstand extreme temperatures, for example in terrestrial volcanic waters or on the ocean floor. I think this is how the patient has been able to survive. These organisms can go into a sort of hibernation until the return of the physical conditions in which they can survive. But the combination of environmental factors that keep them alive is very complex and has yet to be discovered.

Participant: I think we have done enough eviscerating (as opposed to dissecting). Can we take a break?

Participant: To say eviscerating instead of dissecting makes me think of Antonino Ferro's book *The Viscera of the Mind*,[12] and in fact that's the territory we are in with this patient.

Report on the work done by the "group session"

Analyst: One might say that initially each of us struggled to accept this "cerebral paralysis" in the sense of paralysing within ourselves what we already know, and thus in a way regressing to "patient" status in order to meet the patient. As therapists, the loss of spatial-temporal order disorientates us, at least initially, and we search for a point of reference to which to cling. We attempt to create order out of chaos by using the categories of setting and the lack of relatedness because of skipped sessions. This approach may well be valid, but the purpose of this group has been to try to explore beyond the known. Shortly afterwards, we broke out of this impasse, and the group has since made many observations that have stimulated reflections on technique. Initially, we focused on the speed at which the patient narrated events and the therapist read. Speed went from being a disturbing factor, a simple smokescreen, to having a different meaning. It was suggested that speed also serves to cope with or fill a void. During this part of the meeting, the group began to explore form rather than content. In order to make sense of the chaos and the speed of the less effective communicative exchanges, the group concentrated on "specific details".

You said that this patient should be handled and breathed in delicately like a rose (referring to roses brought in by a participant). The patient is extremely fragile, as indicated by the misreading of the word "studies" as "suicide". Several images emerged as the group sought to transform the initial feeling of disorientation; the pinball machine, the courtship dance and Picasso's faces.

The group got in touch with difficult-to-master aspects such as deformity and acting out. What language do we need to learn to transform these aspects?

A first technical suggestion was to listen in the same way as we would listen to a rap song or to seek a more corporeal rhythm of dialogue, like a dance. As therapists, what rhythm do our words need to have in order to convey signals of deep caring, and for us to be therapists rather than physicians? The group explored art in terms of composition in space within the setting – a living composition and on more than one occasion raised the question of how to achieve a spatial closeness that comes closer to the kind achieved in art than to pre- established norms.

Lastly, there was the evocation of extremophilic micro-organisms that sleep for years until changes in the environment allow them to come back to life.

[Two participants intervene]

Participant: Sleeping Beauty is woken up by a kiss.

Participant: Primitive states of the mind are hard to reach: if therapists are too intense, severe patients get upset and withdraw; if they are too distant, they are not reawakened.

Analyst: In fact, we specifically asked ourselves how to enter into the lives of others and, in particular, of such fragile people.

You evoked the song "Good evening doctor",[13] in which a request for love is mixed with intrusiveness and falsification.

How does one keep to the side, engage with pathological aspects of functioning and put them together like Picasso? How does one achieve the necessary oscillation between rigour and fluidity?

The group has shown itself able to resort to diagnostic categories that take a snapshot of the patient's current condition, instead, attempting to maintain an exploratory attitude towards the unknown (Sara-Sarà, meaning "she/he/it will be" in Italian).

The group wonders what the ideal humidity and temperature conditions would be for S. to make transformations. Humidity is also a critical consideration in both fresco and oil painting. This metaphor considers the notion that representation can come about through tangible things: humidity, rhythm, time and composition.

The group made few comments on content, engaging in a tentative exploration of how the technique of child psychoanalysis can be used with severe adults. Metaphors, reveries and associations evoked useful images.

Analyst: The presenting therapist gave an engaging performance: why can't this be done with patients?

Afternoon: the group works on the interaction between the dynamics of the therapeutic couple and the group itself

Participant: There was the Alpine soldiers' festival here in the area, it went on for three days. People welcome them because they have a rather reassuring quality, mind you, some of the things they do are a bit out there, but in a controlled way and legitimised by the institution.

Participant: But what have Alpine soldiers got to do with it now?

Participant: It's quite hard to get started because you have to switch from being a therapist to another role that is not so clear.

Participant: Let's not be like mad patients now!

There is a hard feeling of anxiety and persecution and the analyst decides to intervene.

Analyst: No, it's not a therapy group.

Participant: Speaking of switches, let me tell you something personal. Sometimes it's actually liberating to go to my office because there are times when dealing with everyday life is more tiring than being a therapist.

Participant: Something similar happens in sessions with patients.

I find sessions with a severe patient of mine extremely difficult to bring to a close. She is someone who would never stop; she's like my cat when you try to lift him off the bed and he clings onto it with first one and then both paws; basically, she does the same. On one occasion, while this is happening, the phone rings and I tell her I have to answer it. She prepares to leave, but before going, walks back to the desk and writes a note.

When I finish the next session, I go to read it and find "Put a flower in it".

When I meet with her again, after a short preamble, I tell her that I would like to know more about the note she had left me. She explains that she wanted to suggest that I create something beautiful because they "shit on everything" here. I tell her I am reminded of Sergio Endrigo's song "It takes a flower" and her mention of shit makes me think of De Andrè: nothing grows from diamonds, flowers grow from manure.

The patient then tells me about a truly bizarre dream, and at the end, she says:

"You know, doctor, if someone were to record us (she is obsessed with the idea of being intercepted), they would think we were crazy".

I tell her that since today is a karaoke session, I am put in mind of Bennato and his song "Never Never Land"; we are the ones who can see while perhaps others who believe we are crazy can't.

Participant: We would need to attend a Stanislavski method course. [since some people don't know what it is, the participant explains] It is a famous acting method designed to get actors to make personal identifications with their characters. Some then struggle to return to reality. There occurs a fusion that is difficult to untangle.

Participant: How did Marcello Pesce manage it?

Participant: Who's he?

Participant: [who asks the following question after a bit of stalling within the group] Do you see what it feels like when you don't understand? Now I'll tell you; sometimes, like with today's case, there will be a thousand references that the patient will not help you to understand.

Anyway, he's the main character in the film *Dogman*.

The plot is summarised:

It's about a man (Dogman) living in the suburbs of Rome, an inept man who makes his living dog grooming and dealing heroin on the side. Dogman is harassed by a ruthless and unthinking boss who is hated by all, and who can't be challenged.

Towards the end of the film, this boss commits a crime for which Dogman is held responsible. However, he says nothing, serves his time, and once released, kills the boss.

Participant: What is impressive is the final scene when he has hallucinations, which I saw as the onset of madness.

Participant: I do not see this man as inept; he takes care of his daughter and dogs. Perhaps the inept part is the part that doesn't know how to relate to others. Where you saw hallucinations, I saw something mystical. It is as if he were saying: "Give me recognition because I have done something for you. I have taken upon myself what you are unwilling to allow in; the feeling of being violated, the discouragement, the humiliation". He asks for recognition that has not been or ever will be forthcoming even after the boss's death.

Garrone (the filmmaker) succeeds in giving voice to the senses. There are hardly any dialogues in the film.

Participant: Did you know that the other actors are inmates of Rebibbia prison?

Participant: It didn't win the award for best picture because it was too disturbing.

Participant: There are tolerable situations and then there are those which are far more challenging in that regard. There are times when I feel in danger.

Participant: I saw a documentary where they showed how the mud used to build houses in Africa can contain small invertebrate fish which come back to life when the homes are destroyed by flooding.

Participant: There is hope for us when we get stuck and paralysed in the mud.

Participant: Someone has to kiss you first (with irony).

Participant: Years ago, a particularly strapping man came to see me, and I had the immediate fantasy that if he were to attack me, I would be in trouble. He then started telling me that he had a girlfriend and that he usually fantasised about butchering women to get sexually aroused. After a month and a half of sessions, he tells me he won't be coming again because "I saw that you yawned while I was talking".

Participant: It was the fish's mouth trying to get oxygen.

Participant: But if we suspect a person might commit a crime, the Code of Ethics would allow us to report it.

Participant: It's not a question of the Code of Ethics, it's that when we have to step out of the role of therapists, it's not easy. Look what happens when we have to decide who's going to present the sessions. There is basically a stampede even if we all then have the pleasure of discussing them together.

There is a narcissistic aspect of the therapist's role; it is essential to explore questions about this complex issue.

Report on the "group dynamic"

Analyst: Today we are touching upon sensitive issues without thinking how painful that is. There is the appearance of the trials and tribulations of everyday life and a little paranoid anxiety that expresses itself in the fear of being too disjointed or crazy.

Then there is the aspect of having to deal with our own feelings, which takes work. We feel better behind the label of "doctor". In fact, a somewhat persecutory fantasy of being a patient springs to life. Although not for the first time, the idea of this being a therapy group came up.

What comes across from your words is the issue of closeness and distance, which is of central importance in therapy. May we be in the same shoes as the patient without losing the capacity to think?

The use of songs, "a karaoke session" based on not too verbal a connection seems to offer such potential.

Out of this possibility, the group experiments with feelings such as constriction, submission and revenge and speaks about them throughout the film.

The group experiences the difficulty of losing the narcissistic position and gains insight into the subjective feeling of how difficult it can be to write up sessions and share them with colleagues.

Is there hope for us when we get stuck and paralysed in the mud of overwhelming feeling in the group and with the patient?

It seems that sometimes continuing to speak, maintaining faith in the value of exchanging thoughts and mental pictures and preserving the capacity to be surprised by the other's idea could be enough.

Concluding remarks about group binocular vision

We used the term *binocular vision* to describe a group of therapists' experience as they explored a primitive mode of mental functioning. We hypothesised that what the therapist perceives at this level reflects the difficulty in processing in which the couple have become stuck. This is why the type of difficulty is not made explicit to the group so as to open up the broadest possible field of exploration. The first phase involves turning their gaze towards the therapist-patient couple as two sessions are read and seeking a focus and a transformation of the relational difficulties emerging in the field. We speak here of an interweaving of difficulties experienced by the patient and therapist and by the group.

In the first clinical situation, the crux of the patient's difficulty seems to be the defensive use of splitting. Initially, the group seeks to understand it on an intellectual level, using the theoretical tools they have at their disposal; then, drawing upon the idea of wearing the same shirt as the patient, they focus on how to foster transformations in play.[14] What emerges is the way in which the group advances this transition first through the immersive experience of playing with words and elements such as surprise and fun and the tolerance of the unknown that characterise play.

Through the image of the T-shirt, the group realises the implications of fusion, which is the ability to see how the difficulty that inhabits the therapist-patient couple resides in the group as well. It is in this movement of re-appropriation that a transformational process takes place, as Winnicott described in "The fear of breakdown", but compared to the therapist-patient couple, the group proves to have a greater transformative capacity.

In the afternoon, the group implements stereoscopic vision, i.e. the ability to make self-observations at another level, elaborate some of the dynamics of the group and make connections with the case being presented. When the group struggles to find the link between morning and afternoon, they are faced with a similar problem to the one faced by the patient as she attempts to make sense of complicated feelings and emotions. Hares and crocodiles, the basic assumption fight-flight, become the intermediate area of experience between what is proto-mental and its signification. It is necessary that the group experience the fight-flight basic assumption mode for it to continue to feel contained by its own elaborative capacity.

Proof of the group's continued ability to survive comes from catching the indescribable disaster in advance and transforming it into catastrophic change. There is a struggle between the impulse toward immediate action and creative debate; a struggle to expand rather than explode the mind. For very primitive levels of experience to be encountered and understood, the dream needs to find a place in which it will be welcomed and minds for its transformation: "the somites' dreams need firstly to be felt".[15]

In the second clinical situation, the group confronts primitive emotions that it perceives as analogous to physical deformities. What comes across more clearly in the case of this patient who is in greater psychic distress, is how the lack of distinction between the physical and the psychic characterises the emergence of the proto-mental.

Initially, the group highlights how words can rarely if ever reach these levels of suffering. Next, it explores the physical modalities that can build bridges of communication and allow the therapist to maintain the difficult balance between sharing primitive mental states without being too defensive, so as to foster their transformation. Lastly, the group works on how to establish affective and emotional consonance through such distant modalities of communication as symbolic and protosymbolic, a similar process to the one described by Stern[16] in the primary relationship.

Themes such as falsification, intrusiveness and sometimes the violence with which the patients' sensitive areas are probed are transformed into dreams through cinematographic, pictorial and metaphorical references. In the afternoon, the group feels immersed in the experience of submission, projecting the difficulty regarding the self-imposed working format outward; the group also expresses a fear of sharing too many aspects of madness. The association with the film *Dogman* and with other fragments of personal history (snapshots of experiences with other patients) allows these primitive anxieties to be better addressed to the point of being accepted as human experience among other members of the group.

The numerous references to the arts are not accidental because, as Hans Loewald pointed out as early as 1988, "binocular vision" describes a transformative process that harks back to early developments in the primary relationship. This process is intrinsic to both psychoanalysis and the arts.[17]

The binocular vision that matures in the group, just as it develops physiologically in the individual, functions as a maternal entity that enables the group to perceive itself as a collective entity. It transforms the anxieties that hinder the feeling of oneness and allows the group to open their eyes and see as if for the first time.

Notes

1 The word *idea* is rooted in the Greek etymon "eide", to know, which finds its root in the past tense of the Greek verb "orao", to see.
2 Psychoanalytic insight is about being "able to 'see' meaning" (Bion 1970, p. 223).
3 Bion 1962b, p. 100.
4 Bion 1961, 1962b, 1965, 1970.
5 Bion 1961, vol. 5, p. 113.
6 Bion 1961, vol. 3, pp. 60, 110.
7 Norman and Salomonsson 2005; Lotman 1993; Mason 2000.
8 Kaës 1993, 2010a.
9 Winnicott 1974, 2017d.
10 A participant scrolling through the page numbering reports that he has three identical sheets while one sheet is missing, and the group pauses briefly to rectify this.
11 A. Ferro, *Psychoanalysis and Dreams: Bion, the Field and the Viscera of the Mind*, Routledge, 2014/2019.
12 A song from 1974. In its text, two clandestine lovers are trying to communicate without arousing suspicion in an era before mobile phones and SMS.
13 Ferro 2014; Ferro and Civitarese 2020.
14 Williams 1983, pp. 79–80.
15 Stern 2010; Stern 1985 (In the French edition of the interpersonal world of the infant published on 2010, Stern underlined as in the stratified model of the development, the narrative perspective allow the emergence of the not verbal interactions. "Une conséquence de l'application d'une perspective narrative au non-verbal, telle que ce livre la préconise, a été la découverte d'un langage utile à de nombreuses psychothérapies qui reposent sur le non-verbal." Nahum et al. 1988.
16 Miller 2008.
17 Loewald 1975.

References

Ahumada, J. L. and Ahumada Bush, L. C. (2017), *Contacting the Autistic Child: Five Successful Early Psychoanalytic Interventions*, Routledge, London and New York.

Ahumada Bush, L. C. and Ahumada, J. L. (2005), 'From Mimesis to Agency: Clinical Steps in the Work of Psychic Two-Ness', *International Journal of Psychoanalysis* **86**, 721–736.

Alvarez, A. (1999), 'Frustrations and Separateness, Delight and Connectedness: Reflections on the Conditions Under Which Bad and Good Surprises are Conductive to Learning', *Journal of Child Psychotherapy* **25**(2), 183–198.

Alvarez, A. (2010), 'Levels of Analytic Work and Levels of Pathology: The Work of Calibration', *International Journal of Psychoanalysis* **91**(4), 859–878.

Alvarez, A. and Peltz, R. (2018), 'Conversations with Clinicians', *Fort Da* **24**(1), 66–93.

Amir, D. (2014), *Cleft Tongue: The Language of Psychic Structures*, Routledge, London.

Anagnostaki, L., Zaharia, A. and Matsouka, M. (2017), 'Discussing the Therapeutic Setting in Child and Adolescent Psychoanalytic Psychotherapy', *Journal of Child Psychotherapy* **43**(3), 369–379.

Anzieu, D. (1983), 'Un Soi disjoint, une voix liante: l'écriture narrative de Samuel Beckett', *Nouvelle revue de psychanalyse* **28**, 71–85.

Appelbaum, J. (2012), 'Science and Theory in Modern Physics and Psychoanalysis', *International Forum of Psychoanalysis* **21**, 117–124.

Bancalari, F. (2015), *Fenomenologia e pornografia [Fenomenology and Pornography]*, ETS, Pisa.

Barish, K. (2018), 'Cycles of Understanding and Hope: Toward an Integrative Model of Therapeutic Change in Child Psychotherapy', *Journal of Infant, Child, and Adolescent Psychotherapy* **17**(4), 232–242.

Beckett, S. (1938), *Murphy*, Routledge, London.

Bem, D. J. (2011), 'Experimental Evidence for Anomalous Retroactive Influences on Human Cognition and Affect', *AIP Conference Proceedings,* (Vol. 1408, pp. 191–203).

Bem, D., Tressoldi, P., Rabeyron, T. and Duggan, M. (2016), 'Feeling the Future: A Meta-Analysis of 90 Experiments on the Anomalous Anticipation of Random Future Events', *F1000Research, 4*, 1188.

Benjamin, W. (1997), *Charles Baudelaire: A Lyric Poet in the Era of High Capitalism*, Verso, London & New York, chapter Some Motifs in Baudelaire.

Benjamin, W. (1999), *Little History of Photography 'Selected Writings'*, Harward University Press, Cambridge, MA, London, UK, pp. 514–515, 526–527.

Benjamin, J. (2004), 'Beyond Doer and Done To: An Intersubjective View of Thirdness', *Psychoanalytic Quarterly* **73**(1), 5–46.

Benjamin, J. (2014). Beyond doer and done to: An intersubjective view of thirdness. In *Relational Psychoanalysis* (Vol. 4, pp. 91–130). London and New York: Taylor and Francis.

Bergstein, A. (2018), 'The Psychotic Part of the Personality: Bion's Expeditions into Unmapped Mental Life', *Journal of the American Psychoanalytic Association* **66**(2), 193–220.

Bick, E. (1968), 'The Experience of the Skin in Early Object Relations', *International Journal of Psychoanalysis* **49**, 484–486.

Billow, R. M. (2000), 'Bion's "Passion": The Analyst's Pain', *Contemporary Psychoanalysis* **36**, 411–426.

Billow, R. M. (2003), 'Relational Variations of the "Container-Contained"', *Contemporary Psychoanalysis* **39**(1), 27–50.

Bion Talamo, P. (2011), *Mappe per l'esplorazione psicoanalitica*, Borla, Torino.

Bion, W. R. (1950), *The Imaginary Twin 'Second Thoughts'*, Routledge, London and New York.

Bion, W. R. (1952), 'Group Dynamics: A Review', *International Journal of Psychoanalysis* **33**, 235–247.

Bion, W. R. (1957). Differentiation of the psychotic from the non-psychotic personalities. *Int J Psychoanal*, *38*, 266–275.

Bion, W. R. (1961), *Experiences in Groups*, Tavistock, London.

Bion, W. R. (1962a), 'The Psycho-Analytic Study of Thinking: A Theory of Thinking', *International Journal of Psychoanalysis* **43**, 306–310.

Bion, W. R. (1962b), *Learning from Experience*, William Heinemann, London.

Bion, W. R. (1963), *Elements of Psychoanalysis*, Heinemann, London.

Bion, W. R. (1965), *Transformations*, Heinemann, London.

Bion, W. R. (1967a). The imaginary twin. In *Second Thoughts* (Vol. 1). London and New York: Routledge.

Bion, W. R. (1967b), *Second Thoughts: Selected Papers on Psycho-Analysis*, Heinemann, London.

Bion, W. R. (1970), *Attention and Interpretation: A Scientific Approach to Insight in Pshyco-Analysis and Groups*, Tavistock, London.

Bion, W. R. (1975), *Brazilian Lectures: Rio/São Paulo No 2*, Imago Editora, São Paulo.

Bion, W. R. (1977), *Two Papers: The Grid and Caesura*, Imago Editora, São Paulo.

Bion, W. R. (1979), *A Memoir of the Future, Book 3 The Dawn of Oblivion*, Imago Editora, Rio de Janeiro.

Bion, W. R. (1980). *Bion In New York and Sao Paulo*. (Bion F, Ed.). Perthshire (Scotland): Clunie Press.

Bion, W. R. (1985), *Seminari Italiani*, Borla, Roma.

Bion, W. R. (1991). *A Memoir of the Future, Book 2 The Past Presented. Rio de Janeiro: Imago Editora. [Reprinted in one volume with Books 1 and 3 and 'The Key']*. London: Karnac Books.

Bion, W. R. (1997a), *A Memoir of the Future, Book One: The Dream*, Imago Editora.

Bion, W. R. (1997b), *Taming Wild Thoughts*, Karnac Books, London.

Bion, W. R. (2005), *Italian Seminars*, Routledge, London.

Bion, W. R. (2013), *Los Angeles Seminars and Supervision*, J. Aguayo and B. Malin, eds., Karnac Books, London.

Bion, W. R. (2014), *A Seminar in Paris: Held on July 1978*, C. Mawson, ed., Karnac Books, London.

Bloom, K. (2000), 'Movement as a Medium for Psychophysical Integration', *Free Associations* **8B**, 151–169.

Boccara, P., Gaddini, A. and Riefolo, G. (2009), 'Authenticity and the Analytic Process', *American Journal of Psychoanalysis* **69**, 348–362.

Bollas, C. (1979), 'The Transformational Object', *International Journal of Psychoanalysis* **60**(1), 97, 107.

Bollas, C. (2015), *Being a Character*, Routledge, London and New York.

Bolognini, S. (1994), 'Transference: Erotised, Erotic, Loving, Affectionate', *International Journal of Psychoanalysis* **75**, 73–86.

Bonito Oliva, A. (1984). *Klimt Kokoschka Schiele: Disegni e acquarelli [Designs and Watercolors]*. Milano: Mazzotta.

Bowlby, J. (1979), *The Making and Breaking of Affectional Bonds*, Tavistock, London.

Brady, M. T. (2018), *Analytic Engagements with Adolescents: Sex, Gender, and Subversion*, Routledge, London and New York.

Breslin, J. E. B. (1993). *Mark Rothko: A Biography*. Chicago, IL: University of Chicago Press.

Brokken, J. (2010). *Shpirti baltik. Fate njerëzore në Estoni, Letoni dhe Lituani Albanian*. (Atlas, Ed.). Amsterdam.

Brusset, B. (2012), 'The Therapeutic Action of Psychoanalysis', *International Journal of Psychoanalysis* **93**, 427–442.

Bucci, W. (1985), 'Dual Coding: A Cognitive Model for Psychoanalytic Research', *Journal of the American Psychoanalytical Association* **45**, 155–187.

Bucci, W. (1997), *Psychoanalysis and Cognitive Science: A Multiple Code Theory*, Guilford Press, New York.

Butler, J. (1990), *Gender Trouble: Feminism and the Subversion of Identity*, Routledge, London and New York.

Cartwright, D. (2010), *Containing States of Mind: Exploring Bion's Container Model in Psychoanalytic Psychotherapy*, Routledge, London and New York.

Caldwell, L. (2007) Being and sexuality: Contribution or confusion? In: Caldwell, L. (ed.), Winnicott and the PsychoanalyticTradition. London: Karnac.

Cartwright, D. (2016), 'A Bionian Formulation of Shame: The Terror of Becoming One's Self', *International Journal of Psychoanalysis* **3**, 1–29.

Chodorow, N. J. (1989), *Feminism and Psychoanalytic Theory*, Yale University Press, New Haven, CT.

Civitarese, G. (2013), *The Inaccessible Unconscious and Reverie as a Path of Figurability*, H. B. Levine, G. S. Reed and D. Scarfone, eds., Routledge, London, chapter Truth and the Unconscious in Psychoanalysis, pp. 220–239.

Civitarese, G. (2014), 'Between "Other" and "Other": Merleau-Ponty as a Precursor of the Analytic Field', *Fort Da* **20**, 9–29.

Collovà, M. (2007), *Sognare l'analisi*, Boringhieri, Torino, chapter Per una psicoanalisi sostenibile [For a Sustainable Psychoanalysis].

Comini, A. (2018). Dessin: la ligne de vie d'Egon Schiele. In *Egon Schiele, Fondation Louis Vuitton* (Éditions G). Paris.

Corbett, K. (2011), 'Gender Regulation', *Psicoanalytic Quarterly* **80**, 441–459.

Corbett, K. (2014), 'The Analyst's Private Space: Spontaneity, Ritual, Psychotherapeutic Action, and Self-Care', *Psychoanalytic Dialogues* **24**, 637–647.

Cresti, R. and Nannini, N. (2014), *Passaggio a Krumau: Omaggio a Schiele [Journey to Krumau: Homage to Schiele]: Catalogo della mostra personale [Catalogue of the Personal Exhibit]*, Centroffset, Reggio Emilia.

Danckwardt, J. F. and Wegner, P. (2007), 'Performance as Annihilation or Integration?', *International Journal of Psychoanalysis* **88**, 1117–1133.

de Heredia, J. M. (1893). *Les Trophées*. Paris: A. Lemerre.

De Toffoli, C. (2014). *L'esperienza della psicoanalisi*. (B. Bonfiglio, Ed.). Milano: Franco Angeli.

Demaria, C. (2004), 'The Performative Body of Marina Abramović: Rerelating (in) Time and Space', *European Journal of Women's Studies* **11**, 295–307.

Derrida, J. (1996), *Résistances de la psychanalyse*, Galilee, Paris, chapter Etre juste avec Freud – L'histoire de la folie l'ÿge de la psychanalyse (confrence prononce le 23 novembre 1991).

Dimen, M. (2003), 'Keep On Keepin' On: Alienation and Trauma Commentary on Ruth Fallenbaum's Paper', *Studies in Gender and Sexuality* **4**, 93–103.

Dimen, M., & Goldner, V. (2002). *Gender in Psychoanalitic space: between clinic and culture*. New York: Other Press.

Dodds, E. R. (1951). *The Greeks and the Irrational*. Berkeley, CA: University of California Press.

Dodds, E. R. (2009), *I greci e l'irrazionale*, Einaudi, Torino.

Durban, J. (2014), 'Despair and Hope: On Some Varieties of Countertransference and Enactment in the Psychoanalysis of ASD (Autistic Spectrum Disorder) Children', *Journal of Child Psychotherapy* **40**, 187.

Eco, U. (1964), *Apocalittici e integrati: Communicazione di massa e teorie della cultura di massa*, Bompiani, Milano.

Edwards, B. (1981), *Drawing with the Right Brain*, Souvenir Press, London.

Eiguer, A. (1997a). *Le générationnel*. Paris: Dunod.

Eiguer, A. (1997b). Transgénérationnel et temporalité. *Revue Française de Psychanalyse*, *61*, 1855–1862.

Eiguer, A. (2004), *L'inconscient de la maison*, Dunod, Paris.

Eshel, O. (2017), 'From Extension to Revolutionary Change in Clinical Psychoanalysis: The Radical Influence of Bion and Winnicott', *Psychoanalytic Quarterly* **86**(4), 753–794.

Eshel, O. (2019), *The Emergence of Analytic Oneness: Into the Heart of Psychoanalysis*, Routledge, London and New York.

Faimberg, H. (1988), 'The Telescoping of Generations: Genealogy of Certain Identifications', *Contemporary Psychoanalysis* **24**, 99–117.

Fallaci, O. (1975), *Lettera ad un bambino mai nato*, Rizzoli, Milano.

Ferro, A. (2002), 'Narrative Derivatives of Alpha Elements: Clinical Implications', *International Forum of Psychoanalysis* **11**, 184–187.

Ferro, A. (2006), 'Clinical Implication of Bion's Thought', *International Journal of Psychoanalysis* **87**, 989–1003.

Ferro, A. (2008), 'Book Review: A Beam of Intense Darkness by James S. Grotstein', *International Journal of Psycho-Analysis* **89**, 867–888.

Ferro, A. (2009), *Mind Works: Technique and Creativity in Psychoanalysis*, Routledge, London and New York, chapter Psychosomatic Pathology or Metaphor: Problems of the Boundary, pp. 73–106.

Ferro, A. (2011), *Avoiding Emotions, Living Emotions*, Routledge, London and New York.

Ferro, A. (2014). *Le viscere della mente Sillabario emotivo e narrazioni*. Milano: Raffaello Cortina.

Ferro, A. (2017), 'The Pleasure of the Analytic Hour', *Italian International Annual* **11**, 67–78.

Ferro, A., & Molinari, E. (2018). The Analyst as Dreaming Filmmaker. In C. Bonovitz & A. Harlem (Eds.), *Developmental Perspectives in Child Psychoanalysis and Psychotherapy*. London and New York: Routledge. https://doi.org/10.4324/9781351235501

Ferro, A. and Basile, R. (2009), *The Analytical Field: A Clinical Concept*, Karnac Books, London.

Ferro, A., & Civitarese, G. (2015). *The Analytic Field and Its Transformations. The Analytic Field and Its Transformations*. London: Karnac Books. https://doi.org/10.4324/9780429481048

Ferro, A., & Civitarese, G. (2020). *Vitalità e gioco in psicoanalisi*. Milano: Raffello Cortina.

Feyerabend, P. (1993), *Against Method*, Verso, London.

Fischer, W. G. (1996). *Egon Schiele, 1890–1918: Pantomima di lussuria, visioni di mortalità [Pantomime of Luxury, Visions of Mortality]*. Koln: Taschen.

Fogassi, L. and Ferrari, P. F. (2007), 'Mirror Neurons and the Evolution of Embodied Language Current Directions', *Psychological Science* **6**, 136–141.

Fonseca, V. R. (2006), 'Self, Other and Dialogical Space in Autistic Disorders', *International Journal of Psychoanalysis* **87**, 439–455.

Fornari, F. (1982). Dall'esperienza naturale di bellezza alla fondazione psicoanalitica dell'estetica. In L. Russo (Ed.), *Estetica e psicologia*. Bologna: Il Mulino.

Fraiberg, S., Adelson, E. and Shapiro, V. (1975), 'Ghosts Nursery A Psychoanalytic Approach to the Problems of Impaired Infant-Mother Relationships', *Journal of the American Academy of Child Psychiatry* **14**, 387–421.

Frege, G. (1988), *Ricerche logiche [Logical Investigations]*, Guerini e Associati, Milano.

Freud, S. (1905), 'An Outline of Psychoanalysis', *Standard Edition* **23**, 139–207.

Freud, S. (1909), 'Family Romances', *Standard Edition* **9**, 235–242.

Freud, S. (1940), 'Three Essays on the Theory of Sexuality', *Standard Edition* **VII**, 123–243.

Freud, A. (1954), 'The Windering Scope of Indication for Psycho-Analysis', *Journal of the American Psychoanalytic Association* **2**, 607–620.

Gedo, J. E. (1983), *Portraits of the Artist: Psychoanalysis of Creativity and Its Vicissitudes*, Routledge, London.

Giannachi, C., Kaye, N. and Shanks, M. (2012), *Archaeologies of Presence: Art, Performance and the Persistence of Being*, Routledge, London.

Glenberg, A. M. and Gallese, V. (2012), 'Action-Based Language: A Theory of Language Acquisition, Compre Hension, and Production', *Cortex* **48**, 905–922.

Glover, N. (2009), *Psychoanalytic Aesthetics: An Introduction to the British School*, Karnac Books, London.

Goldstein, G. (2013). *Art in Psychoanalysis: A Contemporary Approach to Creativity and Analytic Practice*. London: Karnac.

Goodman, S. (2017), 'The Balancing Act: Concurrent Parent-Child Work', *Journal of Infant, Child, and Adolescent Psychotherapy* **16**(4), 252–257.

Grinberg, L. (1985). Bion and Group Psychotherapy. In M. Pines & P. Kegan (Eds.) (pp. 176–191). New York: Routledge.

Grotstein, J. S. (2007), *A Beam of Intense Darkness*, Karnac Books, London.

Grotstein, J. S. (2013). The Psychoanalytic Covenant Human Sacrifice as the Hidden Order of Transference Countertransference. In R. Oelsner (Ed.), *Transference and countertransference today*. London and New York: Routledge.

Grubbs, F. E. (1950), 'Sample Criteria for Testing Outlying Observations', *The Annals of Mathematical Statistics* **21**(1), 27–58.

Harris, A. (1997), 'Beyond/Outside Gender Dichotomies—Introduction: New Forms of Constituting Subjectivity and Difference', *Psychoanalytic Dialogues* **12**, 1001–1017.

Harris, A. (2002). Minds and Dialogues in Analytic Spaces—Negotiating Certainty and Uncertainty: Reply to Commentary. *Psychoanalytic Dialogues*, (12), 1001–1017.

Harris, A. (2011). The Tavistock Model Paper on Child Development and Psychoanalitic Training. In M. Harris, E. Bick, M. Harris, & W. Harris (Eds.) (pp. 25–43). London: Karnack.

Hartman, J. J. (2018), 'Risk Factors in Suicide: Mark Rothko and His Art', *Journal of Psychiatric and Mental Health* **3**(2), https://doi.org/10.16966/2474-7769.127.

Hegel, G. W. F. (1975), *Aesthetics: Lectures on Fine Art*, Clarendon Press, Oxford.

Herman, J. (1997), *Trauma and Recovery*, Basic Books, New York.

Hinshelwood, R. (2016). Containing primitive emotional states: approaching Bion's later perspectives on groups. In H. Levine & G. Civitarese (Eds.), *The W.R. Bion Tradition: Lines of Development* (pp. 407–419). London: Karnac.

Hockney, D. (2001), *Secret Knowledge: Rediscovering the Lost Techniques of the Old Masters*, Thames & Hudson, New York.

Horney, K. (1942). *The Collected Works of Karen Horney* (Vol. II). New York: W. W. Norton & Co.

Houzel, D. (1997). *Thinking: a dialectic process between emotion and sensations*. Lanham, Maryland: Jason Aronson Inc.

Imbasciati, A. (2004), 'A Theoretical Support for Transgenerationality', *Psychoanalytic Psychology* **21**, 83–98.

Isaacson, W. (2011), *Steve Jobs*, Little, Brown Book Group, London.

Kaës, R. (1993), *Le groupe et le sujet du groupe: Eléments pour une théorie psychanalytique du groupe*, Dunod, Paris.

Kaës, R. (1994), *La parole et le lien: Les processus associatifs dans les groupes*, Dunod, Paris.

Kaës, R. (1998), 'L'intersubjectivité: un fondement de la vie psychique', *Repères dans la pensée de Aulagnier Topique* **64**, 45–73.

Kaës, R. (2009a), 'La rèalité psychique du lien', *Le Divan familial* **22**, 109–125.

Kaës, R. (2009b), *Les alliances incoscientes*, Dunod, Paris.

Kaës, R. (2010a), *L'appareil psychique groupal*, Dunod.

Kaës, R. (2010b), *Transmission de la vie psychique entre générations*, R. Kaës, H. Faimberg, M. Enriquez and J.-J. Baranes, eds., Dunod, chapter Introduction au concept de transmission psychique dans la pense de Freud.

Kant, I. (1781), *Critik der reinen Vernunft*.

Katz, W. W. (2016), 'The Experience of Truth in Psychoanalysis Today', *Psychoanalytic Quarterly* **85**, 503–530.

Kernberg, O. (1999), 'Psychoanalytic Psychotherapy and Supportive Psychotherapy: Contemporary Controversies', *International Journal of Psychoanalysis* **80**, 1075–1091.

Klein, M. (1932), *The Psycho-Analysis of Children*, Humanities Press, New York, NY.

Klein, M. (1955), *Envy and Gratitude and Other Works, 1946–1963*, Delacorte Press/Seymour Lawrence, chapter The Psychoanalytic Play Technique: Its History and Significance, pp. 122–140.

Knafo, D. (2012), *Dancing with the Unconscious: The Art of Psychoanalysis and the Psychoanalysis of Art*, Routledge, London.

Knowlson, J. (1996), *Damned to Fame: The Life of Samuel Backet*, Bloomsbury Publishing, London.

Korbivcher, C. F. (2005), 'The Theory of Transformations and Autistic States: Autistic Transformations: A Proposal', *International Journal of Psychoanalysis* **86**, 1595–1610.

Kuhn, T. S. (1962), *The Structure of Scientific Revolutionary*, University of Chicago Press.

La repubblica (1981), "Sarà sempre Odissea (It will be *Odyssey* forever)". In it Italo Calvino presented to the public a new version of the *Odyssey* printed by Valla Foundation-Mondadori.

Lafarge, L. (2008), 'On Knowing Oneself Directly and Through Others', *Psychoanalytic Quarterly* **77**, 167–197.

Landi, A. (2000), 'Optical Illusions', *Art News* **99**, 134–141.

Langer, S. (1953), *Feeling and Form: A Theory of Art*, Scribner, New York.

Laor, I. (2007), 'The Therapist, the Patient, and the Therapeutic Setting: Mutual Construction of the Setting as a Therapeutic Factor', *Psychoanalytic Dialogues* **17**(1), 29–46.

Lehman, S. (1999), *The Tibetans: A Struggle to Survive*, Virgin, London.

Levine, G. S., Reed, H. B., & Scarfone, D. (2013). *Unrepresented States and the Construction of Meaning Clinical and Theoretical Contributions*. London and New York: Routledge.

Loewald, H. W. (1975), 'Psychoanalysis as an Art and the Fantasy Character of the Psychoanalytic Situation', *Journal of the American Psychoanalytic Association* **23**, 277–299.

Lombardi, R. (2008), 'The Body in the Analytic Session: Focusing on the Body-Mind Link', *International Journal of Psychoanalysis* **89**, 89–109.

Lombardi, R. (2016), *The Bion Tradition*, H. L. Levine and G. Civitarese, eds., Routledge, London, chapter The Hat on the Top of the Volcano: Bion's O and the Body-Mind Relationship, pp. 223–238.

Lombardi, R. (2017), *Body-Mind Dissociation in Psychoanalysis: Development After Bion*, Routledge, London.

López-Corvo, R. E. (2002). *The Dictionary of the Work of W. R. Bion. Bion.* London and New York: Routledge.

Lotman, J. M. (1990). *Universe of the Mind A Semiotic Theory of Culture*. Bloomington, Indiana: Indiana University Press.

Lotman, J. M. (1993). *La cultura e l'esplosione*. Milano: Mimesis.

Malerba, L. (1997), *Itaca per sempre*, Mondadori, Milano.

Marks-Tarlow, T. (2015), 'Commentary on Dynamical Systems Therapy: Theory and Practical Applications', *Psychoanalytic Dialogues* **25**(1), 131–135.

Mason, A. (2000), 'Bion and Binocular Vision', *International Journal of Psychoanalysis* **81**, 983–988.

Matte-Blanco, I. (1988), *Thinking, Feeling, and Being: Clinical Reflections on the Fundamental Antinomy of Human Beings and World*, Routledge, London.

Mauk, M. D. and Buonomano, D. V. (2004), 'The Neural Basis of Temporal Processing', *Annual Review of Neuroscience* **27**, 307–340.

Mawson, C. (2019), *Psychoanalysis and Anxiety: From Knowing to Being*, Routledge, New York.

McKinley, B. D., Brown, E. and Caldwell, C. H. (2012), 'Personal Mastery and Psychological Well-Being Among Young Grandmothers', *Journal of Women & Aging* **24**(3), 177–193.

Migliozzi, A. (2016). The W. R. Bion Tradition. In H. L. G. Civitarese (Ed.) (pp. 315–326). Karnac.

Miller, J. D. (2008), 'Loewald's "Binocular Vision" and the Art of Analysis', *Journal of the American Psychoanalytic Association* **56**(4), 1139–1159.

Milner, M. (1950), *On Not Being Able to Paint*, Heinemann Educational Book, London.

Mitrani, J. (1998), 'Never Before and Never Again: The Compulsion to Repeat, the Fear of Breakdown and the Defensive Organization', *International Journal of Psychoanalysis* **79**, 301–316.

Molinari, E. (2014). Action across emptiness. *Journal of Child Psychotherapy*, *40*(3), 239–253.

Molinari, E. (2016), *The Wilfred Bion Tradition*, H. B. Levine and G. Civitarese, eds., Karnac Books, chapter Communicating Pictures: Aesthetic Aspects as a Developmental Tool for the Contained-Container Interaction, pp. 489–500.

MOLINARI, E. (2017). *Field Theory in Child and Adolescent Psychoanalysis*. London and New York: Routledge.

Nahum, J. P., Harrison, A. M., Lyons-Ruth, K., Morgan, A. C., Bruschweilerstern, N., Tronick, E. Z., Stern, D. N. and Sander, L. W. (1988), 'Non-Interpretive Mechanisms in Psychoanalytic Therapy: The "Something More" than Interpretation', *International Journal of Psychoanalysis* **79**, 903–921.

Norman, J. (2004), 'Transformations of Early Infantile Experiences', *International Journal of Psychoanalysis* **85**, 1103–1122.

Norman, J. and Salomonsson, B. (2005), ''Weaving Thoughts': A Method for Presenting and Commenting Psychoanalytic Case Material in a Peer Group', *International Journal of Psychoanalysis* **86**(5), 1281–1298.

Novick, K. and Novick, J. (2013), 'Concurrent Work with Parents of Adolescent Patients', *Psychoanalytic Study of the Child* **67**, 103–136.

Obholzer, A. (1996). Psychoanalytic contributions to authority and leadership issues. *The Leadership & Organization Development Journal*, *17*(6), 53–56.

Ogden, T. H. (1985), 'The Mother, the Infant and the Matrix: Interpretations of Aspects of the Work of Donald Winnicott Contemp', *Contemporary Psychoanalysis* **21**, 346–371.

Ogden, T. H. (1989), 'On the Concept of an Autistic-Contiguous Position', *International Journal of Psychoanalysis* **70**, 127–140.

Ogden, T. H. (1996), 'Reconsidering Three Aspects of Psychoanalytic Technique', *International Journal of Psychoanalysis* **77**, 883–899.

Ogden, T. H. (1997), 'Some Thoughts on the Use of Language in Psychoanalysis', *Psychoanalytic Dialogues* **7**, 1–22.

Ogden, T. H. (1999), ''"The Music of What Happens" in Poetry and Psychoanalysis', *International Journal of Psychoanalysis* **80**, 979–994.

Ogden, T. H. (2001), 'Reading Winnicott', *Psychoanalytic Quarterly* **70**(70), 299–323.

Ogden, T. H. (2004). On holding and containing, being and dreaming. *International Journal of Psycho-Analysis*, *85*, 1349–1364.

Ogden, T. H. (2007), 'On Talking-As-Dreaming', *International Journal of Psychoanalysis* **88**, 575–589.

Ogden, T. H. (2017), 'Dreaming the Analytic Session: A Clinical Essay', *Psychoanalytic Quarterly* **86**(1), 1–20.

Ogden, T. H. (2019), 'Ontological Psychoanalysis or "What Do You Want to Be When You Grow Up?"', *Psychoanalytic Quarterly* **88**(4), 661–681.

Pallasma, J. (2005). *The eyes of the skin*. Chichester, England: John Wiley & Sons Ltd.

Pasche, F. (2010). Reading French Psychoanalysis (pp. 694–765). London and New York: Routledge.

Piontelli, A. (1989), 'A Study on Twins Before or After Birth', *International Review of Psychoanalysis* **16**, 413–426.

Piontelli, A. (2002), *Twins: From Foetus to Child*, Routledge, London and New York.

Pistiner de Cortiñas, L. (2009). *The Aesthetic Dimension of the Mind: Variations on a Theme of Bion*. London: Karnac Books.

Placanica, A. (1993), *Storia dell'inquietudine: metafore del destino dall'Odissea alla guerra del Golfo*, Donzelli, Firenze.

Privitera, G. A. (2005). *Il ritorno del guerriero. Lettura dell'Odissea*. Einaudi.

Reiner, A. (2010). Primitive mental state: A psychoanalytical exploration of the origin of meaning. In Van Buren J & Alhanati S (Eds.). London: Routledge.

Rhode, M. (2011). The 'autistic' level of the Oedipus complex. *Psychoanalytic Psychotherapy*, *25*(3), 262–276.

Rizzolatti, G., Fadiga, L., Gallese, V. and Fogassi, L. (1996), 'Premotor Cortex and the Recognition of Motor Actions', *Cognitive Brain Research* **3**(2), 131–141.

Ross, C., ed. (1990), *Abstract Expressionism, Creators and Critics*, Abrams Publishers, New York.

Rothko, C. (2004). *The Artist's Reality: Philosophies of Art by Mark Rothko*. New Haven, CT: Yale University Press.

Rothko, M. (1957), 'Interview', *The New Yorker* **74**, 26–33, 103.

Rothko, M. (2006). *Writings on Art*. (M. Lopez-Remiro, Ed.). New Haven, CT: Yale University Press.

Saj, A., Fuhrman, O. and Vuilleumier, P. (2014), 'Patients with Left Spatial Neglect also Neglect the "Left Side" of Time', *Psychological Science* **25**, 207–214.

Saketopoulou, A. (2014), 'Mourning the Body as Bedrock: Developmental Considerations in Treating Transsexual Patients Analytically', *Journal of the American Psychoanalytic Association* **62**(5), 773–806.

Salomonsson, B. (2006), 'The Aesthetic Dimension of the Psychoanalytic Process', *Scandinavian Psychoanalytic Review* **29**, 2–12.

Salomonsson, B. (2007), 'Talk to Me Baby, Tell Me What's the Matter Now', *International Journal of Psychoanalysis* **88**, 127–146.

Salomonsson, B. (2012), 'Has Infantile Sexuality Anything to Do with Infants?', *International Journal of Psychoanalysis* **93**(3), 631–647.

Salomonsson, B. (2014), 'Psychodynamic Therapies with Infants and Parents: A Critical Review of Treatment Methods', *Psychodynamic Psychiatry* **42**(2), 203–223.

Salomonsson, B. (2015), 'Therapeutic Action in Psychoanalytic Therapy with Toddlers and Parents', *Journal of Child Psychotherapy* **41**(2), 112–130.

Sartre, J.-P. (2004), *The imaginary: A Phenomenological Psychology of the Imagination/ Jean-Paul Sartre; Revisions and Historical Introduction by Arlette Elkanm-Sartre; Translation and Philosophical Introduction by Jonathan Webber*, Routledge, London.

Scarfone, D. (2015), *The Unpast: The Actual Unconscious*, Karnac Books, London.

Schopp, C. (2018), *L'origine du monde: Vie du modèle*, Phébus, Parigi.

Schröder, K. A. (2000). *Egon Schiele e la "finis Austriae*. Milano: Skira.

Segal, H. (1991), *Dream, Phantasy and Art*, Tavistock/Routledge, London.

Sender, L. G. (1994). *Reading Freud's reading*. New York: New York University Press.

Sequeri, P., ed. (2009), *Il corpo del "logos": pensiero estetico e teologia cristiana*, Glossa, Milano.

Simões, L. and Passos, M. C. (2018), 'The Performance Art of Marina Abramovic as a Transformational Experience', *Psychology* **9**, 1329–1339.

Stefana, A. and Gamba, A. (2018), 'From the "Squiggle Game" to "Games of Reciprocity" Towards a Creative Co-Construction of a Space for Working with Adolescents', *International Journal of Psychoanalysis* **99**(2), 355–379.

Stern, D. N. (1985), 'The Interpersonal World of the Infant: A View from Psychoanalysis Developmental Psychology', *International Journal of Early Childhood* **19**(1), 73.

Stern, D. N. (2003). *Le monde interpersonnel du nourrisson Une perspective psychanalytique et développementale*. Paris: PUF.

Stern, D. N. (2010). *Forms of vitality: Exploring dynamic experience in psychology, the arts, psychotherapy, and development*. Oxford University Press.

Stewart, H. (2003), 'Winnicott, Balint, and the Independent Tradition', *American Journal of Psychoanalysis* **63**(3), 207–217.

Tricomi, F. (2001). *Estetica e psicoanalisi [Aesthetics and Psychoanalysis]*. Soveria Mannelli (CZ): Rubbettino.

Tustin, F. (1972), *Autism and Childhood Psychosis*, Hoghart, London.

Tustin, F. (1987), *Autistic Barriers in Neurotic Patients*, Karnac Books, London.

Tustin, F. (1994a), 'Autistic Children Who are Assessed as Not Brain-Damaged', *Journal of Child Psychotherapy* **20**, 103–131.

Tustin, F. (1994b), 'The Perpetuation of an Error', *Journal of Child Psychotherapy* **20**, 3–23.

Ubaldo, N. (2000), *Atlante illustrato di filosofia*, Giunti Editore, Firenze.

Weil, S. (1949), *L'enracinement: Prélude à une déclaration des devoirs envers l'être humain*, Gallimard, Paris.

Whitefield, C. and Midgley, N. (2015), '"And When You Were a Child?": How Therapists Working with Parents Alongside Individual Child Psychotherapy Bring the Past Into Their Work', *Journal of Child Psychotherapy* **41**(3), 272–292.

Williams, M. H. (1983), '"Underlying Pattern" in Bion's Memoir of the Future', *International Review of Psychoanalysis* **10**(1), 75–86.

Williams, M. H. (2010), *The Aesthetic Development: The Poetic Spirit of Psychoanalysis Essays on Bion, Meltzer, Keats*, Karnac Books, London.

Williams, P. (1999), '"Non-Interpretive Mechanisms in Psychoanalytic Therapy" by Daniel Stern et al. and What Is "Applied" in "Applied" Psychoanalysis? by Aaron H. Esman', *International Journal of Psychoanalysis* **80**, 197–210.

Winnicott, D. W. (1945), 'Primitive Emotional Development', *International Journal of Psychoanalysis* **26**, 137–143.

Winnicott, D. W. (1954), *Through Paediatrics to Psycho-Analysis*, Brunner/Routledge, London, cap XII.

Winnicott, D. W. (1969), 'The Use of an Object and Relating Through Identifications', *International Journal of Psychoanalysis* **50**, 711–716.

Winnicott, D. W. (1971a), *Playing and Reality*, Basic Books, Inc., New York, chapter Transitional Objects and Transitional Phenomena (1951), pp. 1–25.

Winnicott, D. W. (1971b), *Playing and Reality*, Basic Books, New York, chapter Playing: A Theoretical Statement, pp. 38–52.

Winnicott, D. W. (1971c), *Playing and Reality*, Penguin Books, London.

Winnicott, D. W. (1974), 'Fear of Breakdown', *International Review of Psychoanalysis* **1**, 103–107.

Winnicott, D. W. (1989a), *Elements in Psycho-Analytic Explorations*, D. W. Winnicott, R. Shepherd and M. Davis, eds., Harward University Press, London, chapter On the Split-off Male and Female (1966), pp. 168–189.

Winnicott, D. W. (1989b), *Psycho-Analytic Explorations*, D. W. Winnicott, R. Shepherd and M. Davis, eds., Kamac Books, chapter The Fate of the Transitional Object in Psycho-Analytic Explorations (1959), pp. 53–58.

Winnicott, D. W. (2007). *Winnicott and the Psychoanalytic Tradition: Interpretation and Other Psychoanalytic Issues* (caldwell L). London: Karnac

Winnicott, D. W. (2017a), *The Collected Works of D. W. Winnicott Volume 3, 1946–1951*, L. Caldwell and H. Taylor Robinson, eds., Oxford University Press, London.

Winnicott, D. W. (2017b), *The Collected Works of D. W. Winnicott Volume 5, 1955–1959*, L. Caldwell and H. Taylor Robinson, eds., Oxford University Press, London.

Winnicott, D. W. (2017c), *The Collected Works of D. W. Winnicott Volume 6, 1960–1963*, L. Caldwell and H. Taylor Robinson, eds., Oxford University Press, London.

Winnicott, D. W. (2017d), *The Collected Works of D. W. Winnicott Volume 11, Human Nature and The Piggle*, L. Caldwell and H. Taylor Robinson, eds., Oxford University Press, London.

Index